Sandplay in Three Voices

Sandplay in Three Voices provides a unique and engaging understanding of sandplay – a growing modality of psychotherapy. Emerging out of informal conversations among three senior therapists, it examines the essential aspects of sandplay therapy as well as the depth and breadth of the human psyche.

The book is organized into eight sections covering eight of the most important topics in sandplay – Therapist, Silence, Child, Mother, Self, Shadow, Chaos, and Numinous. Each section begins with a trialogue discussing the theory, history and practice of sandplay in that area. The trialogues allow the reader to witness three senior therapists addressing and attempting to understand the many layers of each topic, and reflect their agreements and disagreements as they reveal their individual thoughts on, and personal experiences of, the themes they discuss. Each trialogue is followed by a set of solo presentations in which each author focuses on her contribution, and on the role of each topic in sandplay.

Illustrated by original clinical examples, this unique approach addresses issues of concern to analysts and other psychotherapists. Its basic orientation makes it of particular value in the study, practice and teaching of sandplay therapy.

Kay Bradway, PhD, is a founding member of the C.G. Jung Institute of San Francisco and of the International Society of Sandplay Therapy, and co-founder of Sandplay Therapists of America. She is co-author of two books on sandplay.

Lucia Chambers, MA, is co-founder and currently educational consultant of Sandplay Therapists of America. She is known for her research on the archetypal feminine and the Black Madonna.

Maria Ellen Chiaia, PhD, is a Jungian analyst and a teaching member of the international and national societies of Sandplay Therapy and is currently board chair of the national society in the USA. She is an international lecturer and author of numerous publications.

Sandplay in Three Voices

Images, Relationships, the Numinous

Kay Bradway, Lucia Chambers and Maria Ellen Chiaia

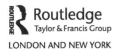 Routledge
Taylor & Francis Group

LONDON AND NEW YORK

First published 2005 by Routledge
27 Church Road, Hove, East Sussex, BN3 2FA

Simultaneously published in the USA and Canada
by Routledge
711 Third Avenue, New York, NY 10017, USA

Routledge is an imprint of the Taylor & Francis Group, an informa business

Typeset in Times by RefineCatch Ltd, Bungay, Suffolk
Cover concept by Lucia Chambers and Charlotte M Turner,
graphic design by Sandra Heath

British Library Cataloguing in Publication Data
A catalogue record for this book is available from the British Library

Library of Congress Cataloging in Publication Data

Bradway, Kay, 1910–
Sandplay in three voices : images, relationships, the numinous / Kay
Bradway, Lucia Chambers, Maria Ellen Chiaia.
    p.   cm.
  Includes bibliographical references and index.
  ISBN 1–58391–729–2 (hardback : alk. paper)
  1. Sandplay. 2. Psychotherapy. I. Chambers, Lucia. II. Chiaia,
Maria Ellen. III. Title.
  RC489.S25B725 2004
  616.89′1653–dc22   2004018528

ISBN 1-58391-729-2 (hardback)
ISBN 13: 978-1-58391-729-9

Contents

Illustrations

FIGURES

PLATES

These plates are intended to give the reader a sense of how each of the eight topics might look in a sandtray. They were selected from Lucia Chambers' collection. Except for the first plate, Therapist, they are not referred to in the text.

1   Therapist
2   Silence
3   Child
4   Mother
5   Self
6   Shadow
7   Chaos
8   Numinous

Foreword

Thomas Singer

This is a book by three women who have shared a calling to practice the art of sandplay therapy. They also clearly love theory and, like the alchemists of old, their work and art are a complex mix of theory and practice. Engaging in either theory or practice alone automatically invites the other to be considered. The authors have chosen a unique way in which to discuss their theory and practice. They have created their own sandplay in words in which they make a "tray" together by engaging in a "trialogue" and then they break down the "trialogue" by each making her own word "tray" based on her individual reactions to the preceding "trialogue." It makes for a rich brew, well worth working through carefully as it is filled with practical information and deep wisdom.

In first plunging into the material of this book, I was reminded of a "trialogue" that I attempted with two friends 35 years ago. The three of us were in our final year of medical school and we sat down one evening with a tape recorder in an effort to debrief one another about what had most impacted us in our then short but intense medical studies. Our talk was mostly filled with our shared anxiety and horror at having been exposed to such a large daily dose of physical and emotional suffering. We were very new to the art and practice of medicine, so that what comes through in a rereading of the transcript of that youthful exchange is our seriousness, the depth of our calling, and our inexperience. In this book, three mature women engage in a similar "trialogue" – but only after each has practiced her art for many years. What comes through in this "trialogue" is their seriousness, the depth of their calling, and their experience. What links the two "trialogues" is the fact that people don't bother to take note of such conversations unless what they have to say is incredibly important to them and they have a "calling" to pass it on to others.

Two other associations link the "trialogue" of my memory with this "trialogue." There are lots of "mm-hmm," "yep," "yup," or "that's right" and similar grunts of affirmation in this manuscript, as there were in the tape-recorded conversation with my medical student colleagues. It is hard to make these utterances of visceral agreement come alive in a transcript – but I know from my own experience that each "mm-hmm" is an important, if somewhat awkward, cue to the reader that what is being said strikes a deep and resonant chord in the listener, as it should in the reader. Pay close attention to the "mm-hmms" in this manuscript. They signal that a chord of important, shared experience is being struck.

The other thing that came to mind as an associational link between the two "trialogues" is the almost Easter-egg-like thrill of the hunt for "pearls." As medical students, we used to walk around with our small black books in which we would write down "pearls." "Pearls" were those incredibly useful bits of practical clinical wisdom that one couldn't find anywhere other than on the wards, trailing around behind attending physicians. "Pearls" were the gems that older, more experienced clinicians had gleaned from years of practice and would pass on or "drop" as they made their rounds. It occurs to me that this is a book of sandplay therapy "pearls." They are dropped at unexpected moments and often catch the reader unsuspecting, such as an apparently spontaneous and unplanned "trialogue" about where sandplay therapists should best position themselves during the session. Again, I would advise the reader to keep an eye out for the "pearls" that are being rather casually dropped along the way in this book and can easily be missed. In fact, the best analogy that has come to my mind in trying to place this book in context for the reader is to think of it as akin to the "pearl" books we kept as medical students that gathered in one place all the elusive but essential gems of knowledge that one needs to survive in the survival business – but, in this case, the pearls being offered are of the highest grade. This is not a "how-to-conduct" sandplay therapy book; this is not a book about technique; this is a sandplay therapy "pearl" book.

A final reflection/association on the nature of this book. As I was reading the manuscript, the word *therapeutae* kept coming to mind. I couldn't remember who or what the "therapeutae" were – but I kept thinking to myself, the authors of this book are *therapeutae*. So I did a search on the *therapeutae* and found reference to them in an ancient text, *De Vita Contemplativa*, attributed to Philo Judaeus and written in *c.* 30 CE:

> They are called *therapeutae* and *therapeutrides*, either because they profess an art of medicine more excellent than that in general use in cities (for that only heals bodies, but the other heals souls which are under the mastery of terrible and almost incurable diseases, which pleasures and appetites, fears and griefs, and covetousness, and follies, and injustice, and all the rest of the innumerable multitude of other passions and vices, have inflicted upon them), or else because they have been instructed by nature and the sacred laws to serve the living God, who is superior to the good, and more simple than the one, and more ancient than the unity with whom, however, who is there of those who profess piety that we can possibly compare? Can we compare those who honor the elements, earth,

water, air, and fire? To whom different nations have given names, calling fire *Hephaestus*, I imagine because of its kindling, and the air *Hera*, I imagine because of its being raised up, and raised aloft to a great height, and water *Poseidon*, probably because of its being drinkable, and the earth *Demeter* because it appears to be the mother of all plants and of all animals.

The therapeutic sect of mankind, being continually taught to see without interruption, may well aim at obtaining a sight of the living God, and may pass by the sun, which is visible to the outward sense, and never leave this order which conducts to perfect happiness. But they who apply themselves to this kind of worship, not because they are influenced to do so by custom, nor by the advice or recommendation of any particular persons, but because they are carried away by a certain heavenly love, give way to enthusiasm, behaving like so many revelers in bacchanalian or corybantian mysteries, until they see the object which they have been earnestly desiring.

So, this is a modern book by three women who, like the contemplative *therapeutae* of ancient times, share a calling – as sandplay therapists. They are passionate, knowledgeable and still asking all the important, basic questions about their theory and practice. Their questions and continuing curiosity about their calling should not be taken as a questioning or doubt about the value of their tradition. They "know" it is a good and valuable work, and this book reflects the depth of their care and knowledge of their calling.

Acknowledgments

Our gratitude centers on our teacher and mentor, Dora M. Kalff. It was she who started each of the three of us in different ways and at different times on our journeys that eventually led to the writing of this book. She has been therapist, teacher, mentor and colleague. What a magical way she had of combining theory, wisdom and inspiration!

Many colleagues have encouraged us in our writing of this book. We want to especially express our appreciation for the encouragement and help of John Beebe and Harriet Friedman.

Our heartfelt thanks go to Joyce Camuyrano Cunningham, who edited all of the chapters and assisted us in diverse other ways – always with good cheer. We think of her as a teammate.

Our greatest thanks go to the many sandplayers whose processes contributed to our learning, to our reverence for the human psyche, and now to this book.

Thank you all.

Kay, Lucia, Maria

Introduction

Kay Bradway

This book is not a "how-to-do-it" book on sandplay. How to do sandplay has been covered by several other authors, including Dora Kalff (1980, 2003), who developed sandplay therapy and founded the International Society for Sandplay Therapy, and Estelle Weinrib (1983) and Kay Bradway (with Barbara McCoard, 1997) who were co-founders of Sandplay Therapists of America.

Nor does this book give a background or history of the development of sandplay. This is covered in a book by Rie Rogers Mitchell and Harriet Friedman (1994).

No, this book is not concerned with the practice or history of sandplay. It is concerned with some of the basic elements of sandplay therapy, in fact of all depth therapies, which we have struggled to understand more fully. Therapists who do not use sandplay will find our explorations and struggles compatible with some of their own queries and experiences. Jungian therapists will find familiar references and a familiar language. Jung was the one who stimulated Dora Kalff's development of sandplay therapy. It was when she was incorporating what she had learned from Margaret Lowenfeld's teaching of Sand Worlds that Kalff realized the extent to which clients' series of sandtrays followed the process of what Jung had identified as individuation. Jungian principles were used by Kalff throughout the development of sandplay. Sandplay is a nonverbal therapy using sandtrays, water and miniatures provided by an empathic therapist who encourages the making of anything one wants in the tray without interventions or interpretations. Verbal therapy is used as an adjunct to sandplay, or sandplay as an adjunct to verbal therapy, but the two are kept separate from each other, even, in certain circumstances, being done by two different therapists.

This book evolved out of informal conversations with each other about different aspects of sandplay. It became clear to us that an underlying aspect that has not received the attention it deserves is the importance of relationship in sandplay. There is, of course, the relationship between the therapist and client. But also there is the relationship of each to the sand; of each to their own unconscious and to the other's unconscious; the relationship to the unlived side of the shadow of each; the relationship to the numinous, the spiritual, to something beyond each where the Self connection is made between the two.

We wanted to get at the meaning of some of these connections. Not just a single meaning, but the many deep meanings; meanings that were personally important to each of us. We began to appreciate that our understanding of the basics of all depth therapies was being stimulated by our conversations and our mutual explorations. Our commonalities were valued, but our differences were enlivening. Along the way it occurred to us that it might be helpful to others to see, to experience, some of our deliberations. Perhaps we should collaborate on a book.

To test the waters of collaboration the three of us put on a panel on sandplay at the 2001 Conference of the Division 39 of Psychoanalysis of the American Psychological Association in Santa Fe. In giving entirely separate presentations, we found that we not only respected each other's differences but learned from them.

Deciding which of many topics to concentrate our attention on posed an initial problem. We were particularly focused on the universal importance of relationship in many topics. But our guidelines were not rigid. The final selection of topics to receive our focus was narrowed down to: therapist, silence, child, mother, Self, shadow, chaos, numinous. To share our actual process, we taped our conversations about each of these topics. Our editing of the transcribed conversations was done jointly and consisted mainly of deleting excessively repetitive statements and off-the-track ramblings. Our three-way dialogues, which we came to identify by the more descriptive "trialogues," show our struggles in addressing and attempting to understand the essence and the many layers of each topic. They reflect our agreements and disagreements as we reveal our individual thoughts and personal experiences.

As we proceeded with this project, we recognized we are quite different from one another, with an age range of 40 years, with diverse family and religious backgrounds, with differences of style in writing. Our important commonalities are our several years of Jungian analysis and our individual excitement at the time we were introduced to sandplay therapy: Kay's "I was totally turned on," after experiencing a presentation by Dora Kalff of the sandplay process of a young child; Lucia's "It was heaven," when her analyst introduced her to using sandplay as an adjunct to the verbal analysis; Maria's "The creative, silent parts of me felt seen and held and found a place for expression."

Our initial enthusiasm for sandplay was heightened by our many years of employing sandplay in our own therapeutic work, both with children and with adults.

To highlight our differences in style, in experiences and in approach to each of the eight topics, we decided to include individual contributions by each of us to follow each of the eight trialogues. We did not compare notes about what we were writing until the completion of our individual contributions on each topic. And then we read them aloud. We were gratified by how different each was from the others in style and content and yet how well the three seemed to fit together.

Writing this book has been an experience in self-exposure, in letting down our hair. We have let ourselves ask naive questions akin to the child's universal question: "Is there a Santa Claus?" We have okayed our giving far-out answers. We have thought small and we have thought big. We have shown our familiarity with the writings of others and have referred to the theories of accepted authorities. But we have not been bound by any authority except by the mercurial one in each of us.

Part I

Therapist

Chapter 1

Therapist trialogue

LUCIA: Sometimes I wonder who is the client, because the interaction and what happens in the trays are just as challenging and transforming for me. And the client does not seem to notice anything, but I am sure going through a lot. Sometimes there is an interchange of energy; and sometimes, there may be transformation or shifting in the psyche. I really wonder if they are there for me or I if am there for them.

KAY: Both. That is a good point, though.

LUCIA: So that means the therapist has to be open to the same transforming energy and shadow stuff as the client. Or maybe more, do you think?

KAY: Well, you can't just say, "I'm going to be more open." Or, "I'm going to be related to my shadow."

LUCIA: You either are, or you're not.

KAY: That is the reason we have so much training: for people to learn how to do sandplay because it is very hard. You don't talk so you can't cover up. Just like with children, you can't cover up things, they seem to know. When you get related, then you can't cover up. And, if you haven't had enough training yourself and therapy yourself, you're thinking and feeling things that you don't even realize the client may pick up.

MARIA: When we trained in sandplay, I never liked the idea of the witness, that we are witnessing the sandplay process. This idea never really fit for me because we are impacted by feelings and body sensations as well as the imagery that appears in the sand. We are not just witnessing; we are fully engaged.

KAY: True.

MARIA: With all of ourselves. We are responding – not only responding to but also being a stimulus to what is created.

LUCIA: "Witness" is kind of impersonal, isn't it?

MARIA: Yeah, too objective or outside of.

KAY: Engagement is like being in the soup together, not just stirring the soup.

MARIA: Right. This reminds me of Jung's *Psychology of the Transference* [Jung, 1966d] where there is an alchemical image of the king and queen getting into the bath together. For Jung the king and queen were the symbolic therapeutic couple. Patient and therapist are in the soup together – the bath.

KAY & LUCIA: Mm-hmm.

MARIA: They are both naked, then they merge together and then separate out. But first, when they are both naked, one can feel both of them in it together, both vulnerable and both being transformed. This reminds me of something Jung said, analysis or therapy does not start until the patient has become a problem for the therapist.

KAY: I don't know that.

LUCIA: You don't?

MARIA: You don't know if you agree with that.

KAY: Well, it seems that it could be that an untrained therapist who was seeing someone for the first time might have a problem more quickly than someone who was very well trained. I wonder, from what Jung said, does the therapeutic process start more quickly for the untrained therapist?

LUCIA: Do you mean the sandplayer brought up your own issues?

KAY: Stimulated and engaged your issues, maybe.

MARIA: Stimulated and engaged us to work with our own unconscious as we are working with the sandplayer.

KAY: Yeah, that's better. That makes sense about the engagement. But for the trained person, the patient might not be a problem for them as soon as for an untrained person. So that is the reason I don't like that word "problem." "Engaged" is better. Engagement can be fully experienced without there being a problem. But the experiencing of a problem always carries with it an engagement.

MARIA: Yes, I like "engaged" too. In *The Psychology of the Transference*, Jung seemed to be struggling with his own issues involving the transference.

LUCIA: And it's a very different way of looking at it than – than Freud did, for example. For Freud, therapists are supposed to keep themselves totally out of their emotional responses to the client. But we're not talking only about being emotionally responsive either. We're talking about some other kind of connection.

MARIA: That is fine but I would not want to take the emotions out of it.

LUCIA: The emotions are a signal that something else is going on. It is a symptom or a –

KAY: Sign.

LUCIA: A sign. Yeah, a road marker.

KAY: Well, I was thinking that, when therapy first started, with Janet, for instance, the relationship with the patient was one of curing the patient of pathology. The therapist in those early days used hypnosis to change the patient. I understand that Jung, in the early stage, also used hypnosis. And then he wanted to be completely away from the patient because of

Freud's influence, I suppose. And so he even had patients write down their dreams and not give them to him, so he'd be more out of it.

LUCIA: Huh!

KAY: And it wasn't until later that he became the way that, I think, most analysts operate now, which is to engage and let the engagement go without either hypnotizing or being out of it completely.

LUCIA: So the engaging, the being engaged, how or where does the engagement happen? Does it happen on the feeling level? Does it? What is happening in this engagement?

KAY: I don't know whether you call it feeling or what, but the guts –

LUCIA: The diaphragm, the guts – the *hara*?

KAY: Yes, the Japanese word is *hara*. That's where the real engagement is, and the head may be involved in that, but the *hara*, that is where the deep engagement is. But you don't get that right away, although with some clients you may get it more quickly.

LUCIA: Mm-hmm.

KAY: It's due to transference. The client reminds you of someone and that's just pure transference. And you like them and so you get engaged more easily maybe. Or you may not like them.

LUCIA: So, are we talking about transference? Is it the same thing?

KAY: No, it isn't the same thing. I use the word "co-transference." I think "co-relationship" is probably better. "Co-transference" was only used because people were using the term "transference/countertransference" and I wanted to make it just "co-transference."

LUCIA: Mm-hmm. Mm-hmm.

KAY: The transference is there, but the relationship is more than just transference.

MARIA: Well, that fits with the modalities of thinking right now, getting out of the transference/countertransference dichotomy. Steven Mitchell and others have started a whole school of relational psychology [Mitchell, 1993]. And in sandplay therapy we are also focused on the relationship between the therapist and sandplayer.

KAY: The mother–child relationship is the first relationship that a person has and then, later, the sexual relationship. There are many other relationships, but these are the two maybe prime relationships that come into the patient–therapist relationship.

MARIA: Which two? Mother–child?

KAY: Mother–child and the sexual relationship.

MARIA: Lovers.

KAY: There is also the sibling relationship, but that's different. The parent – the mother–child – is the first. And, in therapy, you do get an erotic relationship many times. It might be necessary for this erotic feeling to constellate. And the handling of these feelings takes a tremendous amount of experience. And some people don't want to talk about it.

LUCIA: Mm-hmm.

KAY: I have found that the erotic feelings may exist for same gender or opposite gender. It's often there.

MARIA: I guess what you're saying is that there are the feelings of this kind.

KAY: That's true. But there is the need for the recognition of those feelings and the handling of them. And that's one of the reasons I think sandplay is so helpful because these feelings can be handled, and often are, in the sandtray.

LUCIA: In the sand.

KAY: Without your having to engage in sexual talk or explanation.

LUCIA: When intimacy is present on an ego level, then you get into problems. What are you going to do then? But if the intimacy, or the relationship, is on another level, it can have a whole different impact on the psyche of both the client and the therapist.

MARIA: So what level are you talking about?

LUCIA: That's what we keep talking around.

MARIA: Well, my first thought was that the connection is symbolic, but it's not just symbolic.

LUCIA: No, it's real.

MARIA: Because it's a real relationship. There is a *you* and there is a *me*: there are the two of us and we are in a real relationship.

LUCIA: Yeah. I wonder if it isn't some kind of an experience of the Self. There is a coming together of who the client is and who the therapist is and there is an acknowledgment of some kind of completeness or place of meeting.

KAY: Or potential for completion.

LUCIA: Yes, that! There is a feeling of totality –

KAY: Of wholeness.

LUCIA: Of wholeness. Yes. So I would think that, on a non-ego level, there could be a profound spiritual union, or a potential or a sense of possibility within the relationship.

KAY: It is very exciting. Sometimes it makes the therapy go. But it can be very dangerous.

LUCIA: How can it be dangerous?

KAY: If therapists aren't sufficiently experienced, their feelings are in danger of being acted on or they may turn the feelings into rejection of the patient. In sandplay there is a protection from this.

LUCIA: That's right.

KAY: I know this from experience. People have come to me for analytic work after they have been severely hurt because the previous therapist was not able to handle their own sexual feelings. I don't find this in sandplay. I don't think I've ever known or heard of it.

LUCIA: And yet there's a love.

KAY: Oh, yes.

LUCIA: And that is felt by both.

KAY: Yes, and it's played out symbolically in the tray, and both know it. The therapist knows when this is going on and the patient knows it.

LUCIA: Yeah.

KAY: But it's distanced.

MARIA: It's distanced but yet we are deeply engaged in feeling the depth of that connection.

KAY: Would you say that again? I think that's important.

MARIA: I said that it's a distant connection in that it is being played out in the sand but we are impacted by and with the sandplayer. We are feeling it deeply with them as they are experiencing it. And we are experiencing with them the feeling of connection, union, and love.

LUCIA: That's why I wonder if it's some aspect of the Self.

KAY: Because it's an experience of wholeness.

MARIA: It is, then. Definitely.

KAY: Yes.

MARIA: Yeah, union. I think about it in terms of a meeting at the level of the Self.

KAY: And the therapist has to be able to recognize this in the tray and not be threatened by it.

LUCIA: Or see it when it isn't there. That is the value of consultation.

KAY: Yeah. And in consultation I have heard people say they have erotic feelings and talking about it in a contained place helps.

MARIA: We also have to look at the negative side of this love connection. If you have that intense feeling of love and merger, you may also – probably will have – intense hatred and rage.

KAY: Yes, rage.

MARIA: All of the developmental issues that were not resolved in the early relationship with the mother will certainly be there.

KAY: And with the lovers.

MARIA: And with the lovers. You also get both the love and the hate.

KAY: Yeah. That's very important.

LUCIA: Are you talking about from client to therapist or therapist to client?

KAY: Both ways.

MARIA: Both ways. I have hated clients.

KAY: I have found it's easier to hate a client when you're not having to respond with words.

MARIA: Right. You just let the feeling move through you.

KAY: You look at them. You look at the images in your head because you aren't playing it out in the tray.

LUCIA: No, you get that anger in the sand.

KAY: If they're not improving, sometimes you do. And if they don't pay their bills and they come late.

MARIA: Or if you are working with trauma and abuse of any kind. Of course you get that anger, and destructive rage will come up.

LUCIA: Or if it seems as if they are putting all of my figures in the sand.

KAY: Yes.

MARIA: Or every time they make a sandtray, they're dumping sand on the floor.

LUCIA: Maybe the sand makes it easier for us to stay deep, and allows us not to come back up to the ego level where we may be scared and angry and feel as if we want to act out these feelings. If we are experienced in that deep place and can stay down rather than think that we personally, our personalities, are involved in this. They're not. The clients don't hate us. There's hate in the room.

MARIA: And you begin to experience this intense feeling as archetypal, so much bigger than both of you.

LUCIA: And if you bring it to the personal level, then they will, too. If you can stay down in that deep place then clients are not going to project as easily on you because you're with them.

MARIA: Although it is my experience that in doing sandplay therapy, you have to work on the ego level as well but you do this in the talk therapy which is an adjunct to the sandplay therapy. The hate must be brought into relationship, out of the archetypal, and humanized between you. Words are necessary to help metabolize these destructive forces. Kalsched's work on trauma [Kalsched, 1996] is a helpful resource to understand the necessity of humanizing these destructive forces of anger and rage.

LUCIA: Exactly. But that means therapists have to be conscious of which level they are working on. Don't you think?

MARIA: You keep bringing this up, Lucia, and I tend not to think about different levels. It is helpful to differentiate when I am working with archetypal material and when I am working with ego or more personal material. Although I don't think they're separate. I don't want to make a split between them, because they are connected.

LUCIA: No, they're not split but they're –

MARIA: Maybe it's foreground and background, because you as the therapist might be working on the foreground of the ego, dealing with the therapy bill, but you know there is this deeper level at work simultaneously.

LUCIA: Yes, but you still keep working on that bill.

MARIA: You're working here but knowing that there's this whole other psychological issue the bill is connected with.

LUCIA: And you're not taking the bill issue personally, as if clients don't like you or you are a bad therapist. Beyond the bill issue or whatever is at the surface, there are other meanings to which the therapist must also attend. When I am doing sandplay training or classes, people sometimes ask, "Don't you ever take anything back into the verbal therapy?" My answer is that you don't take the meaning of specific figures into the verbal therapy, but you take the idea of what's going on.

KAY: You're more aware of these deeper meanings and they enter into the verbal therapy that is done separately.

LUCIA: Yes.

KAY: You've had a verification of your feeling that maybe they are angry at you and, if they don't pay their bill, they probably are angry.

LUCIA: Yes.

MARIA: But maybe they are paying their bill and then you see that a witch is pointing her finger at you.

KAY: Yeah, sure. Sometimes clients pay their bills even when they hate you.

LUCIA: Sure.

MARIA: So then you might see it in the sand.

KAY: But you have to be sure that the witch isn't someone else and not you.

LUCIA: That's right.

KAY: You have to attend to all these things and that's the reason we need verbal therapy that is separate from the sandplay. It is a difficult differentiation for many people to get as to how you separate the two, the verbal part and the sandplay part. I think this is something that non-sandplay therapists bring up. What do you do? And it's different, isn't it, for different people?

MARIA: What Lucia was saying is very helpful, which is that we don't talk about the specific figures but we get the idea of the themes or range of the material that the client is working in. And maybe we've picked it up in the verbal therapy as well or maybe not. Then we begin to find ways to talk about it as it becomes more available to the client. That's important too, because if the material is too unconscious, we don't want to just go for that material either. I wait for it to come up through a dream, or by behavior, or through a feeling in the room.

KAY: Right.

LUCIA: No, but you can kind of lead or ease the client into that area. If you have the sand telling you that there is some witchy energy somewhere with this perfect person that you're talking to, who is very happy and everything is wonderful, you can begin to look for where that witchy energy is. So where is the witch?

KAY: You need a verification of that so you aren't just fishing.

LUCIA: You have to be very skillful, I think, to keep it down there so you don't become the witch.

KAY: And recognize when you are becoming the witch.

LUCIA: Yeah. It's easy to become the witch. The sand is helpful, particularly with adults abused as children.

KAY: Yeah. They can play it out so you can actually see it. That's right.

LUCIA: You do not have to become the recipient of so much rage. The sand just absorbs it.

KAY: Or they can do it right away by symbols in the sand.

LUCIA: I am most grateful for the sand because there is so much rage. And I know that if there were no sand, that rage would come to me eventually.

KAY: Sure. It would have to.

LUCIA: And I really would rather it not. The burying, the smashing – all that comes out.

MARIA: Chaos.

LUCIA: Oh! And the pain, all comes out in the sand, and I don't have to hold it in. But I hold them – while they're going through that.

KAY: But you can hold them so much more easily and with so much more love than if they're directing it at you.

LUCIA: Yeah. The elemental energies that would be very difficult for the therapist to hold in verbal therapy, like sex and rage –

MARIA: Intense love is sometimes hard for clients to let you hold. Sometimes feelings of intense love are frightening.

KAY: Of course.

MARIA: Because it's something they've never had before. Or they've had it and been abused around it or have been violated in some way. The sandplay is helpful here too.

KAY: They can feel protected and more at ease, doing this in the sand. They don't feel as though they have to inhibit any of the erotic or rage feelings either at a conscious or unconscious level. They can just do it and experience it.

LUCIA: And there's not the issue of trust, either, as there always is with a therapist. Can I trust you –

KAY: To handle this?

LUCIA: That is not the issue with the sand. It's just not there.

KAY: I can love and hate you without being afraid of my feelings, because it is happening in the sand.

LUCIA: That's right.

KAY: It's one of the very important advantages of sandplay therapy.

MARIA: I wanted to come back to the discussion we had about different levels. When training, how do you train to hold the sandplay at this level of depth? I found that if trainees have had an experience of an archetypal level of reality they can hold it at some depth. If they are not aware of an archetypal level they are going to keep things on a personal level. Then all of the sandplay work will be seen through an interpersonal transference which I don't always think is helpful.

LUCIA: If you're not conscious of your unconscious.

MARIA: Of the collective unconscious.

LUCIA: Then you're going to be caught up in the stuff that happens.

KAY: You can't read about it.

MARIA: No, and you don't know how to negotiate the archetypal if you have not had your own experience of the archetypal.

KAY: Well, let's talk some more about other kinds of relationships we are holding.

MARIA: We talked mother–child and lovers. I also think that there is –

KAY: Sibling rivalry?

MARIA: Not just sibling rivalry. There is a sibling quality of relationship, like Kohut defines, in terms of twinship [Kohut, 1993]. It's another form of the transference. It's more of a brotherly/sisterly love that is just as powerful.

KAY: Well, love and hate, don't throw out hate, rivalry and jealousy.

MARIA: True.

KAY: There is the father–child relationship, too. There is a difference between the therapist relating to the client in a mother–child way and a father–child way. The father–child way of relating is an achievement level of relating. As the client comes from the deep analytic work to a new level of wanting to achieve, more of a father–child relationship may be called for.

LUCIA: The sand is the deep, organic place of creation. That is where the old ego dies and then something new is created. A birthing takes place.

KAY: It's true.

LUCIA: So we could say that the mother–child relationship is there in the creation, and the holding and nurturing of that creation.

MARIA: Sometimes I find that when the mother hasn't provided that function, a father figure is providing the holding. A maternal function that the father fills.

KAY: I like the word "nurturing" better than "mother" or "maternal." That way we don't limit it to gender.

LUCIA: This has nothing to do with gender.

MARIA: I think "maternal" is important. It is connected to the mother archetype. There is a relationship to the containing maternal that every human being needs. However, a male or female therapist can carry this maternal function.

LUCIA: However, a woman is biologically set up for creation. It's in her body. So does a woman sandplay therapist instinctively bring that into the process? Well, that's one of the things we can wonder about. Who you are does enter the sandtray, in ways we are not even aware of.

MARIA: Whether it's gender or whatever.

LUCIA: Whatever it is, it is there!

KAY: Okay. Good.

MARIA: What is important is that all of these relationships can be seen and experienced in the sand.

LUCIA: Also, what we know and what we don't know.

MARIA: And what they know and what has been spoken or has not been spoken. When seeing the sand picture you may find out something about somebody that you didn't know. Or they might experience or know something about you that they couldn't possibly know. Like when they pick some figure that has deep meaning for you, or that you are deeply connected with, letting you know how deeply connected they are to you through the figure they have chosen.

KAY: Mm-hmm. The numinous.

LUCIA: Yeah.

MARIA: Yeah, but it is the numinous, in relationship to each other.

LUCIA: Yup, and it's there. And that's the Self.

MARIA: This is an experience for both the therapist and the sandplayer of meeting at the level of the Self.

KAY: That's the level of archetypal connection, and at that level we're all connected.

Chapter 2

Therapist

Maria Ellen Chiaia

There is much for psychotherapy to learn from the relationship between the therapist and the client in sandplay therapy. This relationship to the depths of our beings and the ability to hold open the space for the unconscious to express itself in order for the deepest layers of the psyche to emerge is the ground of sandplay therapy. The sandplay therapist's presence and relationship to these depths provides the basis of sandplay therapy and separates sandplay from other forms of play therapy. The therapist's relationship to the client, the sand, different aspects of her own unconscious, both personal and archetypal, and particularly the relationship between matter and spirit are attended to in sandplay.

"Related" is defined as having close harmonic connection. "Relation" is a quality (as resemblance) predicated on two or more things or parts taken together; connection or a state of being mutually or reciprocally interested. "Relationship" is defined as the state or character of being related or inter-related. So the relationship to the clients includes the therapists' relationship to themselves and the other, to themselves and the sand figures, to the other and the sand figures, and to the connections between all of these and the conscious and the unconscious.

"Connect" or "connection" are also interesting words. Definitions for "connect" include to establish relationship, to join or unite; those for "connection" include coherence, continuity, link; the last of these, interestingly, denotes a means of communication. The sandplayer in the presence of the therapist makes a communication with sand, water and miniatures, which have coherence, and continuity with the wholeness of the human being creating the sand picture. This creation may then resonate with the therapist, making a relationship to the therapist. The communication and connection are held in the relationship to and with the therapist. And the relationship of the therapist to their own experience of these depths is the essence of the sandplay. Therapists must first make a connection to the many levels and hold open a large enough space so that clients can connect to their own deeper layers as well.

In Rilke's ninth sonnet from *Sonnets to Orpheus* (1962, p. 63), he speaks of entering a "dual realm," where "voices become eternal." Rilke is expressing the relationship between the known and the unknown, the finite and infinite, or a human experience of the archetypal. In sandplay we create a space for the archetypal experience to come through into the human realm through sand, water and miniatures and through the relationship to the therapist.

However, this relationship to the therapist is a complex one. The sand-player and the therapist create a field of experience, which includes the personal, cultural, and collective levels of the conscious and unconscious of both the therapist and the client. The field of experience is particular to the therapist and client, and all they bring into the room. Grand and Chiaia have written on this field phenomenon, and call it the "transindividual field" (Chiaia, 1997; Grand, 1999; Chiaia and Grand, 2002). Other writers have referred to this field phenomenon (Schwartz-Salant, 1995b; Stein, 1995b; Jacoby, 1999).

Having experienced a sandplay process, the therapist has tempered or forged a connection to the deepest level of the psyche, to the archetype of the Self, the central organizing principle of wholeness. This lived connection enters the field of relationship. The therapist has learned to live and experience two worlds – the "dual realm" in Rilke's words – and holds this place open for the client. Having made a relationship to this territory, when the client enters these realms and reaches for the Buddha or the crystal ball to go into the center of the tray, the therapist recognizes the numinosity of the moment because the therapist has seen and experienced the numinous Self. And the client feels affirmed by the therapist's knowing and experiencing with them this numinous connection to Self.

In our trying to describe this realm and what the therapist actually does in sandplay therapy, Chambers speaks of the therapist attuning herself to the "heartbeat of the psyche." This statement arose during one of our conversations. The heartbeat of the psyche can be experienced by what Bradway calls "purposeful imaging" (Bradway, 2001), using the magic combination of sand, water and miniatures.

In sandplay it is the task of the therapist to create a container for the clients so that the healing movement of the psyche may unfold. Therapists are more than witnesses; they are actively receptive and participating observers. We, the therapists, are called upon to enter into this relationship with an enormous capacity for empathy, patience, trust, and an inner knowing of the power and depth of the unconscious in both its positive and its negative forms.

Chiaia (1995; Chapter 18 of the present volume) describes a meeting at the level of the Self, where the Self archetype becomes constellated between the therapist and client. The client asked the therapist to confirm this experience by having the therapist sign the drawing, which was a Self drawing that the client had created. When asked about this, the client's response was "I could not have created this drawing without you" (1995). The client was referring to the experience of the field where the unconscious of the client and the therapist met. Not knowledge, not understanding, not the conscious mind, but the unconscious of both client and therapist working in resonance created this drawing. Both client and therapist were listening to the heartbeat of the psyche.

Purposeful imaging creates deep empathic resonances within the therapist (Bradway, 2004). The therapist's responses to the client can include feelings, images, and sensations. Sensations arise within the body of the therapist through all of the five senses, plus intuition, the sixth sense. The sand image takes form within the transindividual field in a relational matrix, which is permeated by the nonverbal experience of the healing potential within the psyche. The role of sandplay therapists is to again hold open the possibility for all aspects and qualities of matter and spirit to emerge: darkness and light, trauma and distress, the divine and ineffable in their many forms and combinations. Sandplay therapists have experienced these expressions in their own sandplay journey and know the power and magic of a shared and contained sandplay process.

Sandplay makes the space for the creation of the experience of the Self. The mystery of the Self appears in all of its forms and over time it becomes the guiding archetype. The therapist contains the sandplayer within a meaningful personal relationship and carries the possibility of the transcendent. When there is the appearance of the image of the Self, it occurs within the interpersonal matrix so there is a meeting at the level of the Self. In sandplay the body and the psyche provide the material for the wisdom of the individual and the mystery of the Self to emerge.

In sandplay we have the creation of the sand picture within this place of meeting between the sandplayer and the therapist. This creation within the interpersonal matrix or co-transference holds open the possibility of the transcendent and sets in motion a process of healing which may also contain some aspects of initiation and/or transformation. Initiation involves rites, which are ordinary acts imbued with divine knowledge or wisdom. Initiatory acts receive and transmit spiritual values and the initiate undergoes rituals that help the individual relate to the social group and the collective unconscious while maintaining their individual identity. Initiation as described by Henderson (1967) allows for the transition from childhood to adulthood and to the eventual experience of the individuation process described by Jung (1967).

So the magical act of playing with sand, water, and miniatures is first and foremost a therapeutic modality that heals, but it also has the potential for becoming an initiatory experience of individuation for the sandplayer. This magical act occurs in a nonverbal, non-interpretive space provided by the therapist. In this space of preverbal experience with the elements of earth and water there is the possibility of experiencing what Kalff (1980) describes as the mother/child unity of the ego/Self or what Kawai (1996) describes as a meditative state where therapist thinks with the *hara*. Whether we liken this to the infant child experience of the primal Self or the adult experience of the ultimate Self (Henderson, 1967), we hold open the possibility for the psychological state of wholeness to emerge and guide.

From the therapist's connection to the Self as the guiding principle, transformation becomes possible. What is meant here by transformation is consciousness of processes that alter Self experience. Sandplay is a process that can alter Self experiences. Consciousness can come at that moment of play or it can come later in dreams, analysis or in the review of the sand images.

From the ground of being of the therapist and the client who meet in the transindividual field, the process of creation of the sandtrays begins. From this ground of being through the individual aesthetic of the sandplayer, many archetypal themes that relate to healing and transformation emerge. There are never two sandtrays that are alike, as the process of growth and individuation is an individual and yet universal experience. Individuation, according to Jung, unites the person to their own unconscious depths (both the personal and collective aspects), as well as connecting the person to interpersonal, social, and cultural forces. The sandplayer in the act of creation through the connection to the therapist learns to remain open to the process of becoming, which is the work of individuation. Individuation involves becoming related to the unconscious parts of one's psyche and being open and engaged with the integration of these parts. Life and development as a process of *becoming* through the relationship between therapist and client is the focus of sandplay therapy.

Chapter 3

Therapist

Kay Bradway

"I learned that I liked myself." This sounds like a simple expression but it is truly profound. Someone I had seen for eight years in analysis was asked several years later by her new partner, "What did you get out of all those years of analysis?" She thought for a few minutes and then, as she wrote me later, she replied, "I learned I liked myself."

The response was not "I learned *to* like myself," which would imply a change in feeling towards oneself, but rather that the liking was already there and was, in effect, "discovered."

Several years ago, when I heard a speaker before an audience consisting mostly of women say, "Every woman has inside her a voice that says, 'You are no good,' " I countered with, "Everyone has a voice inside, sometimes very deep, that says, 'You are very special.' " This is the voice that one needs to learn is there and to connect with, form a relationship with.

When a woman I had seen for several years and I were reviewing her sandplay process, she observed, "It is interesting, I didn't know how much I was 'saying.' And isn't it interesting how well I said it." I knew then she had traveled below the self-deprecating voice she had listened to for so many years to the "You are very special" voice and learned she liked herself after all the years of doubting everything she did.

How does one learn, and experience, that there is a sacred, mysterious, magical connection between the ego "I" and another deep inner God-given, if you will, "I" with which one is born and which one retains through life? One way is through depth psychotherapy.

Ever since there has been a therapy of the psyche, that is, psychotherapy, there has been the question of (problem of) the role of the therapist. How much authority does the therapist assume? In the early days of psychotherapy, hypnotism and catharsis were at opposite ends of the authority role of the therapist. In hypnotism the therapist was in complete control, with clients performing after the session whatever the hypnotist/therapist had suggested that they do, and the client not realizing that the suggestion had come from the therapist.

In catharsis, on the other hand, the client talked and the therapist listened. It was recognized that this was helpful. I recall a time later, with the availability of more sophisticated instruments, that a person could play a recording that fed back the kind of remarks required to keep the person continuing in their solo quest for help. It was soon realized, however, that a live therapist was actually desirable in any kind of therapy.

Freud recognized the extent to which patients "transferred" onto him their past feelings for significant persons in their lives. When they were falling in love with him, or hating him, it was not just the personal relationship with him but the transference onto him of feelings toward previous significant others in their lives. As I understand it, Freud wished to maintain a kind of blank page as far as his own personality was concerned. He sat behind his patients so they could not see him or his expressions and could image him in their own way.

I understand that Jung in the early days used some hypnotism with his patients and then abandoned the authoritative stance that hypnotism required and attempted to stay out of the picture as much as possible. I am told he asked patients to write letters to him that they keep to themselves without showing them to him. This was to help minimize the strength of a live relationship between them. In current Jungian analysis there has been a development in which the feelings of the patient toward the therapist, and of the therapist toward the patient, are used extensively in the healing and individuation process. Analysis of the transference (and countertransference) plays a prominent role in much current Jungian analysis.

In using Tarot cards or the *I Ching*, therapist and client work together in analyzing or understanding the ritualized material. They are looking at the material together and analyzing it together rather than the therapist's dominating the interpretation. This tends to result in less resistance and less dependence on the therapist than when the therapist takes a more authoritative stance.

A client's erotic feelings for the therapist may be necessary for the full development of the liking/loving of themselves. But this is a tricky area which is responsible for many of the treacherous and wounding involvements between therapist and client. Therapists are warned in all schools about the dangers of the "acting out" of their own erotic feelings in the therapeutic container or of condoning it on the part of their patients. It has been my experience that there are fewer dangerous transference failures in therapy with sandplay than in verbal analysis. The absence of the necessity for words more easily avoids the potholes that verbal communication provides. The positioning of a toy gun in the sandtray so it is pointing in the direction of the therapist is as strong a communication as "I hate you." It is experienced by both, but doesn't call for an outward response from the therapist. Likewise, an erotic imaging in the tray involving a figure that has previously been experienced as standing for the therapist is silently acknowledged by both, without the need for interpreting it as transference or attempting to prevent it from being imaged and experienced.

With the introduction of sandplay, then, a new role of the therapist evolved. The therapist plays a crucial role in sandplay, but is more removed from the direct reception of rage and love. The sandplay therapist's role is to provide a protected space for sandplayers to freely experience, to develop and to handle their feelings of rage and love. The sand gets the brunt of the heat and the sand does not talk back. The sandplayer gets to "say" and do whatever the sandplayer wants to "say" and do. It is nonverbal and bypasses words that require dialogue.

Anyone who has tried to do sandplay as a process without the presence of a therapist realizes the necessity of one. A relationship to the therapist is necessary in authentic sandplay. The therapist provides not only a free and protected space but also empathy.

So what is this empathy that the therapist has for the sandplayer? I like the word "cherishment," which is in the title of a 2000 book: *Cherishment, a Psychology of the Heart* by Young-Bruehl and Bethelard. *The American Heritage Dictionary*'s definition of the word "cherish" is "to hold dear, treat with affection and tenderness." "Cherishment" indicates the product or the state of being cherished. What a different meaning this has from the meaning of "intervene," which is so often used in referring to the action of the therapist on the client's process. "Intervene" means to come between; to interfere.

The very word "analyze" seems counter to what healing and transformation ideally might be. "Analyze" is defined in the *American Heritage Dictionary* as "to separate into parts the basic principles in order to understand the nature of the whole." Analysis is the "separation of an intellectual or substantive whole into its constituents for individual study." But what we are looking for in individuation is to reach a wholeness. It would seem desirable for clients to develop wholeness in the way that is specifically right for each of them, since all individuals are unique, and finding their wholeness is a unique journey. The role of the therapist would seem to be to provide the circumstances for maximizing the twin urges toward self-healing and growth in each client's journey toward wholeness.

Chapter 4

Therapist

Lucia Chambers

> The meeting of two personalities is like the contact of two chemical substances: if there is any reaction, both are transformed.
>
> (Jung, 1933, p. 49)

It would be easy to assume that in sandplay, co-transference is not as big or powerful an issue as in traditional "talk therapy." The verbal exchange, with its tangle of words, emotional expressions and projections, requires great expertise and vigilance to unravel, whereas the tray, the sand, the water and the little figures might seem to allow the energies of the unconscious to play, bypassing the ego which busily functions in verbal communications. It might seem as if the sandplay therapist does not have to work quite so hard. It might seem as if the nonverbal play in the sand is a short cut to a deeper level. The ego has been hard at work preserving its illusion. The play steps directly into the nonverbal symbolic world of the client's unconscious, thus avoiding the ego and its fog of complexes and projections. It looks so easy. One client exclaimed in disbelief, "That's all you do? Just sit here and don't say anything?"

In actuality, the cognitive techniques, the theories, and the mental agility that therapists have so carefully focused on during the course of their education are bypassed. Beyond that, what is required in sandplay is the courage to descend into the depths of the human psyche and open its mysteries. Sandplay opens doors into the unconscious that have been barricaded closed against the powerful archetypal energies that lie so deep that they can only be touched symbolically. It is "easy" to assume that it is only the client who is plunged into that dark space where the ego engages in a desperate struggle to maintain itself.

Therapists must be present on that deep level to commit to exploring with clients the hidden mysteries of that space. There must be a willingness to be partners in the *participation mystique*. Therapists must be ready to meet the archetypal forces in their own unconscious which will rise up to meet those in the unconscious of clients. Jung says:

By no device can the treatment be anything but the product of mutual influence, in which the whole being of the doctor as well as the patient plays its part ... Hence the personalities of doctor and patient are infinitely more important for the outcome of the treatment than what the doctor says and thinks.

(1966c, par. 163)

Learn your theories as well as you can, but put them aside when you touch the miracle of the living soul. Not theories but your own creative individuality alone must decide.

(Jung, 1970, p. 84)

The sand, the water, and the miniatures can open the door, and propel *both* the client *and* the therapist into that dark energy field where the archetypes of both psyches will be activated. More important than collecting figures, reading books, and attending classes is the sandplay therapist's *conscious* willingness to make that precarious descent in the service of the Self. Therapist and client are in the stew together! This is a connection that might be shown graphically as a cord from the sand into the lap of the therapist (see Plate 1). It is easy, after studying, experiencing, and consulting, to think that you "know" that the client will benefit by doing sandplay, that the moving of the sand in the tray "means" that the client is descending into the unconscious, that a boat "implies" a journey, that a round shape in the sand "indicates" the Self. Actually, in these situations, the therapist has moved away from meeting the client in the relational field of the unconscious. The therapist has been seduced by the unconscious desire to be the all-knowing, powerful Mother or Father. This inflated identification has the negative effect of creating distance between the therapist and the sandplayer. The inflated therapist is not capable of experiencing the necessary openness and vulnerability for an unconscious to unconscious exchange. By assuming this archetypal role of Great Mother, Great Father, Healer, the therapist projects the child role onto the client. A message is conveyed that the client has a weak ego for which the therapist will compensate. The mysterious, healing energy of the Self has been personalized and is claimed by the therapist's ego rather than being acknowledged in the psyches of both. Tragically, the therapist will not only jeopardize the client's development but also destroy the therapist's potential for transformation in the alchemical vessel and the "stew" of the unconscious. Jung says of this situation:

The patient, by bringing an activated unconscious content to bear upon the doctor, constellates the corresponding unconscious material in him ... Doctor and patient thus find themselves in a relationship founded on mutual unconsciousness.

(1966c, par. 364)

In therapy there is always an energy present which pulls away and avoids that deepest level where the Self resides. The ego throws up one defense after another in order to avoid that space where it will be required to give up its carefully wrought, present structure and die in the service of the Self. The symbolic world of sandplay is therefore threatening to the ego. The symbols speak of what the ego cannot.

A symbol carries multidimensional, unlimited meaning, always just beyond understanding. It carries the totality of both the conscious, external life and the unconscious collective experiences of all humankind. The realm of the symbolic is where the opposites can appear, where the inner relatedness can happen, and therefore is the only place where the transformative function can be activated. It is also where the ego is sacrificed.

The ego's attempt to edge away from this threat can produce long ruminations of past misfortunes, wounds, philosophical rationales, and dictionary interpretations. Confusion may come up over practical matters, such as fee disputes, missed appointments and staying late. The sandplay therapist can unconsciously collude in this avoidance by giving direct advice, forbidding, confronting or placating, or by giving specific meaning to a figure. All of these unconscious maneuvers can result in the destruction of the symbolic field, with its infinite depth and breadth of meaning. They can flatten the symbol into a figure in the sand, and thereby reduce the tension held between the opposites. Reductive statements are an intrusion into the inner space where the tension of opposites holds the potential of trans-formation. This symbolic container is the alchemical vessel – the temenos. It is the responsibility of the sandplay therapist to keep this "free and pro-tected" space safe from nonsymbolic, persona-preserving energies. The therapist must consciously choose to meet the *client-other* at that deep place and synchronous moment where each one of them is both the healer and the one being healed. Sandplay therapists, "knowing the Self" by having had their own sandplay experience, can stand firm in faith when faced with the unknown and provide the containment. As a result a bridge can emerge between the unconscious and the ego. Hillman says, "this love for psyche – and not the analysis of 'transference reactions' – alone resolves the stuck transference" (1972, p. 110). A new level of consciousness can then be experi-enced by both. Professor Kawai (1996) says, "I do nothing. I do nothing." What is done is everything; the surrender to the Self. Jung quotes from an alchemical text: "And take care that thy door be well and firmly closed, so that he who is within cannot escape, and – God willing – thou will reach the goal" (1968a, par. 218).

In alchemy Jung found a historical foundation for his life's work of exploring the human psyche. The concept of individuation and the processes involved in it were found in complex, symbolic form in the alchemical texts. Because the alchemists were diligent recorders of their experiences, they left behind detailed texts dating back to the fourth century

BC, many of which still survive. Jung studied several of them and found parallels between the psychological process of transformation and alchemical symbolism.

The alchemists supposedly started their experiments in an effort to transmute base metals into gold. They believed that there were principles governing the universal order. If these principles could be discovered, and the correct ingredients used in the right combination, then it would be only a matter of following this formula to obtain gold. Through their explorations, their mystical visions, their writings, their cumulative thought and their rituals, these adventurers began to experience changes in their own personalities. These were shifts in their perception of life and their part in it. These changes in personality could be compared, in a symbolic way, to the changes happening to the bits and pieces in their crucibles. The very processes they were using for transformation in the physical world were linked to the transformation in their human psyches. Through a series of symbolic alterations, the gold of perfect knowledge paralleled a change in the human soul. There was a recognition of the union of earthly and heavenly truth, a "oneness" and therefore the sacredness of all existence. An alchemical text says it this way:

Heaven above
Heaven below
Stars above
Stars below
All that is above
Also is below
Grasp this.
And rejoice
        Schwartz-Salant, 1995a, p. 51

Jung says, "Everything that happens, however, happens in the same 'one world,' and is a part of it. For this reason events must possess an *a priori* aspect of unity" (1963, par. 662). The squared circle is an alchemical symbol representing the synthesis of two opposing realities: the circle of the mysterious and the square of concrete matter. Schwartz-Salant believes this is a clear statement of the basis of Jung's view of psychotherapy:

It posits the necessity of both understanding a person's process in terms of causal interactions, whether they stem from childhood or present situations, and linking these processes to their a priori aspect of unity. This is precisely the function of the alchemical *coniunctio*; it resides in a third or 'in-between' space of relations, akin to the alchemical *pneuma*, which links the unitary and discrete, separable, realms.

(1995a, p. 14)

This in-between space where the lapis – the philosopher's stone – or the Self can manifest can be experienced many times in the sandplay room by both client and therapist. There is a deep silence when time seems to pause. There is awe in the presence of numinous creation and experience of the sacred. This surrender to the Self, in the depths of the archetypal realm, requires the courage and commitment of the therapist to carry the fire of love, a transpersonal love of a unity for which one is willing to risk the blackest dark, the *nigredo*.

We are the mirror as well as the face in it.
                                                Rumi, 1995, p. 106

Part II

Silence

Chapter 5

Silence trialogue

KAY: I like the word "silence." It calms me. I like silences. In our work silence is important because it's when we're silent that things can happen. That's the reason I think sandplay is so good. It is nonverbal. When we relate to each other, we're relating not through words but through something deeper.

LUCIA: I wonder why there's so little silence in our lives. I don't know of another therapeutic modality that sponsors silence.

MARIA: Meeting another human being in that place of silence allows for a deeper meeting or a different kind of meeting to happen. And valuing what emerges out of that silence is critical to sandplay.

LUCIA: Without controlling it.

KAY: It's so hard for some therapists to value silence in therapy because one has gone to school for so long and learned so much that it's very hard to sit with someone and not think, "Oh, that's a good idea" and then tell it. Maybe that is why when people learn sandplay, they want to interpret. They get ideas, and it's very hard to keep an idea in without verbalizing it to someone.

MARIA: Now, in Freudian analysis, they did start out with the therapist not being very involved.

LUCIA: And there could be long periods of silence that sometimes drove the client or patient crazy. And other times the therapists would just space out or go to sleep so, you know –

KAY: Yes, that is because the patient and the therapist weren't relating. However, the Freudian and Jungian ideas have changed. Relating to your patient has become important. In the past you were taught to avoid relating, and if you had an erotic feeling toward a patient, that was all wrong. In Freudian psychoanalysis, the therapist was supposed to be a blank screen. In Kalffian sandplay therapy, we think the relationship is *the* most important thing.

MARIA: There is another point about silence I would like to discuss. In classical Freudian theory, silence was seen as a resistance. If you weren't associating, you were resisting. So there was a pressure to speak. The patient was supposed to be free-associating through words. In sandplay therapy one expresses through images; nonverbal images are being expressed in the sand.

LUCIA: In Freudian analysis didn't the analyst sit out of view?

MARIA: Yes.

LUCIA: In sandplay, there's silence but there is a visual relationship. There's the visual relationship to the figures in the sand and there's the visual relationship between the therapist and the client, which creates another kind of relationship. The sandplay therapist isn't absent at all. The therapist is *so* present. To be present in that way requires more than just talking. There's a lot of it that's visual because, now, you're meeting eyes and you're nodding your head. You're not saying anything but there's a sense of being with, huh?

KAY: Yes, but in sandplay, the way I did it, I sat behind the patient.

LUCIA: You did? Dora Kalff sat directly across.

KAY: Yes, I know.

LUCIA: I would look up and –

KAY: You'd relate to her.

LUCIA: I could tell from her face that she was there, with me, in the sand.

KAY: Yes, it's interesting. In a discussion with another sandplay therapist I said that therapists usually sat behind the client but sometimes, they sat across from the client. And the other therapist said, "I don't know any-one that sits across from the patient." So this is an interesting difference, isn't it? Where do you sit, Maria?

MARIA: I sit across, to the side. So I don't sit directly across but off to the right.

KAY: You can see each other though.

MARIA: Yes.

KAY: I defend my sitting behind because it was the only way I could do it in my office. Many of us defend what we do because we have no other way of doing it.

LUCIA: That's right.

KAY: And Dora Kalff had a great big room with enough space to sit wherever she wanted to, and sometimes the patient would go behind and not let her see them. But that was up to them.

MARIA: I have people who will block my vision.

LUCIA: So what's happening, then, in the silence?

MARIA: When you're not seeing what they're doing?

LUCIA: Yeah.

MARIA: You are seeing that there needs to be a space of privacy or a blocking of what is being created.

LUCIA: Then in this instance, the sandplayer and the therapist are seeing the emergence of these energies of the unconscious at the same time.

KAY: Exactly. Even when I was sitting behind the client and we didn't have eye contact, still the two of us were looking at their production together.

LUCIA: At the same time.

KAY: Which is maybe as deep as looking at each other. And so I never felt I wasn't looking at the client because we both were looking at what they were doing. And then there was something more. There was something from guts to guts.

LUCIA: Is the relationship from guts to guts somehow formed through what is happening in the sand, or is the relationship that is happening being held by what is happening in the sand?

KAY: That's the holding place.

LUCIA: So it's an entirely different relationship than it would be if we were talking.

MARIA: Sandplayer and therapist are both being impacted and responding to what's emerging in the sandtray.

KAY: At first it's that, and then it gets deeper, it engages us, guts to guts.

MARIA: And what is happening in this relationship, in and through the silence, begins to resonate between us.

KAY & LUCIA: Yes!

KAY: And something then comes out of that resonance. The sandplay then reflects that something new has happened. Then the real process gets going. But the real process doesn't always happen.

LUCIA: No, it doesn't.

MARIA: So what we are talking about in the sandplay work is about all these different relationships: the relationship to the sand, to the figures, to what's emerging between us. And all these relationships resonate and impact each other.

KAY: The relationship between therapist and sandplayer is a very complex relationship. What's left out of the relationship, until later, are words. They may come in. The sandplayer may talk but I don't encourage it. In most therapies, they would encourage talking. If there's resistance to talking in these other therapies, the therapist is responsible for trying to reduce that resistance. And then you may get antagonism between the two, patient and therapist.

MARIA: Well, I guess that what you're saying is that if you meet that resistance, you get more resistance.

KAY: If you focus on it, sometimes you get more.

MARIA: Rather than allowing for something to emerge that is an unknown to both of you, something creative that is trying to emerge that the client knows nothing about.

KAY: So sandplay therapists encourage silence.

MARIA: Now, children will tell stories and –

LUCIA: So do adults sometimes.

MARIA: But it's not talking on just a conversational level. It's more talking about what's being created or what's emerging or stories, metaphors that are coming from the sandplay.

LUCIA: I'm thinking as you're talking that words actually get in the way of a deeper relationship, a relationship that goes below the ego and below the head. The minute you add words, you bring in the head. And it's all over then as far as I'm concerned. If you bring in the head, you lose the access.

MARIA: But you were also saying that sandplayers may use words to tell stories.

LUCIA: Yes. Or sometimes there are feelings about what's being created.

KAY: I found that in the beginning of doing sandplay, people talk more. I think they felt this was required in therapy.

LUCIA: That in therapy you are supposed to talk.

KAY: And so they would talk some. If they did this for long, I would say something like, "I wonder if you feel that you have to talk." And that may have interrupted the sandplay for a minute and we'd talk a little about that and I'd just say, "You don't have to."

MARIA: I just don't talk back.

KAY: Yes. The talking will drop if you don't talk back. But sometimes it goes on. Sometimes a person has done other sandtray work and they have been asked to tell what everything is. So they think they're supposed to.

MARIA: Sometimes I try not talking, not responding, and if that doesn't work, sometimes I need to say something.

KAY: Mm-hmm. If there's anxiety?

MARIA: Silence is just not familiar. We were talking in the beginning about how silence isn't very prevalent in our culture. And to most people it is not familiar to be with someone and not talk.

LUCIA: Silence doesn't have any credibility. Words have a lot of credibility.

MARIA: Then as sandplay therapists we have to model, either by words or non-verbally, the value of silence and not talking while creating a sandtray.

KAY: Then clients will start to feel another kind of relationship and, when they feel it, then they don't need to talk.

MARIA: As sandplay therapists we are creating a space for something else.

KAY: We're valuing something that –

LUCIA: That's been lost.

KAY: By doing that, we go back, you see, deeper, because, biologically and historically, words came in quite late. Baby and mother relate without words, through feeling and touching. Also, early in the development of the human race, they didn't use words. Now, it's very seldom that people are together without talking, except maybe when they're in love.

MARIA: Yes.

KAY: But when people are not talking and yet communicating, it takes them deeper. That's why in sandplay people go deeper more quickly than they do in talk therapy.

MARIA: I wanted to add something here. In *The Interpersonal World of the Infant* by Daniel Stern, his infant research shows that in early development, the nonverbal communication that goes on between a mother and a baby is a very special time of sharing. And when words do come for both the baby and the mother, this nonverbal connection is lost. During very early development, a different kind of self is developing, in that nonverbal resonance between mother and baby. Through the silence of relationship this resonance may occur between sandplayer and the sandplay and the therapist.

KAY: Yes, that is communication. In a very close love relationship, words are often not necessary. They even get in the way.

MARIA: How much love is a part of that early connection with mother does color all of our later love experiences and what's possible or not. In the sandplay therapy this place may be touched and healed in and through the nonverbal connection to the sand, the figures and the therapist.

LUCIA: I'm thinking of June Matthews' favorite topic, the gaze – the gaze between the mother and the child and the reflection back to the child of love and acceptance through mother's gaze. And then, I'm wondering if we do that in some way when we are looking at the tray and the appearance of the energy that is coming. There is such a mutual admiration going on about what is happening. It's very affirming on a nonverbal level, which is what the mother and child do. And that's what we do in sandplay therapy.

KAY: It's like mirroring, this affirmation of the individual. And that's why it's so important in sandplay to appreciate what the person is doing and not diagnose or evaluate. I've said that so many times but I get so disgruntled when I hear therapists evaluating what a person has put in: "Oh, that means that they're so and so," like they're hungry. Well, I don't think that helps in the relationship. If you appreciate what they're doing and feel that they're trying to do something to help their hunger, then that's affirmation. They're so used to being evaluated. It's nice to be appreciated.

LUCIA: You think silence is as hard for the therapist as it is for the client?

KAY: Maybe harder. I think it's awfully hard.

LUCIA: I do, too.

KAY: But if you've had your own sandplay process, then you know the value of not having someone talk; you know the value of that silence. If you have had that in your own personal experience, that allows you to tolerate the silence as a therapist.

MARIA: I remember my own discomfort with the silence when I began as the sandplayer. But then after a while, through the therapist's modeling, I realized I did not have to understand or talk about the sand scene. I could then let the sand image speak for itself. I began to let it speak to me. I became familiar with that silence through the mirroring of my sandplay therapist. At first I began to feel just comfortable with the silence, and then I began to really relish it.

KAY: Appreciate it.

MARIA: Yes, and then the words began to feel intrusive. When I became the sandplay therapist, I knew the benefits of silence.

KAY: You could trust it.

MARIA: Yes.

LUCIA: My experience of doing sandplay was relief. Because I had been in verbal therapy and I never thought that my words said what I wanted to say. The silence was heaven. And that it was not only okay, but it was what you're supposed to do – not talk. I felt comfortable, and it was okay.

MARIA: I actually had both simultaneously. There was the discomfort, the social pressure to talk. "There's a person there; I'm supposed to talk." But, on the other hand, there was great relief. It is important not to leave that out; another deeper part of me was thinking, "Oh, thank you. I'm going to be met in a different place."

KAY: Well, you felt appreciated for yourself and not for what you were saying. You could just be you, without any verbal response, and still be cared for.

LUCIA: It's a way of dropping off all of those outer confirmations, all the personas, all the parts of a persona – just dropping them away. And you can always pick them up when you leave.

KAY: Yeah, you have to.

LUCIA: It's not like you throw them away. But you can just set them aside for a little bit.

KAY: And no expectations. The therapist isn't expecting anything from you. They're just viewing what you're doing in the sand and – it's always exciting to see what someone does in the sand.

LUCIA: Isn't it!

KAY: And we do not have to know a lot of background.

LUCIA: You know, I tried – I did an experiment, a couple years ago, about not knowing anything about the sandplayer. Age and sex is about all I got. And then they just did sand. And you know what? It didn't matter.

MARIA: I have tried this approach when doing consultation. I'd get the age, sex and the presenting problem.

KAY: Yeah, I've done that, too. When a lot of background stuff is reported, then the viewers tend to start relating to the figures in terms of the background material. They will point out figures in the tray and say, "That's her father." "That's her mother."

LUCIA: That's right, so in order for something else to happen, sometimes I do a group consultation silently. We look at the series of slides of the trays without talking. Then members of the group give responses of "Oooh!" or "Ahhh!" or "what was that?" As we are looking, the energy may be kind of jangly and then a tray comes and everybody says, "Oooohhhh!" And there are no words at all.

MARIA: And the experience of "Ahhhh!" is new to people who have never seen sandplay before. We will be looking at a series, and there may be chaos and disruption and then some kind of organization in the psyche occurs, and there is an aesthetic to it and everyone notices. It reminds me of an idea I found in a book called *Zen and the Art of Motorcycle Maintenance* [Pirsig, 1974]. If a group of people see or hear something that is of quality, everyone in the room will know it. The premise of the book is that everybody knows what quality is. You don't have to have words for it. You experience it. It's a visual, kinesthetic reality. If a group of people see or hear something that is of quality, everyone in the room will know it.

KAY: Better than if they said it in words.

LUCIA: Yes.

MARIA: There is a quality that is recognizable by human beings when there is the appearance of an image of the archetype of the Self.

KAY: And that appearance is due to the relationship that has been going on between the therapist and sandplayer as well as the sandtray. There's a double experience of the Self.

LUCIA: There is an inner recognition of the Self before the words. We tend to want to nail it down with words. We say, "If there's a circular shape in the sand, that's a Self tray." Or "If there's a mandala, that's a Self tray." Well, not necessarily. But then we go at it – we, us wonderful, hubristic, sandplayers want to label and nail it down. The minute you begin defining and nailing down this ineffable thing, you lose it.

KAY: Dora said that the only thing that is universal about Self trays is that there is a numinous experience.

LUCIA: Now we have to struggle to see what this word "numinous" means? I think this is the struggle we have all the time in this kind of work and why we have so much trouble with research, with credibility, with writing, is because words don't do it.

KAY: It's hard to talk about it or write about it because then we have to use words. And you can see it in the trays.

MARIA: Well, I do not want people to get the idea that we never talk. When the client is working in the sand we value silence. At other times we talk. We work with dreams. We work with transference. We do psychotherapy but when the person is doing the tray, we don't talk.

KAY: That's an important point. Sandplay usually takes up only part of the session and the rest may be used for verbal therapy. Or sandplay may not occur at every session and the other sessions are devoted to verbal therapy.

LUCIA: In managed care, everything is diagnoses and words. There's nothing that acknowledges the silence – nothing about that at all. So maybe in doing our work, faith and trust in relationship to silence must come. Trusting that there is another level of psyche operating all the time and it is not acknowledged with the majority of people in the psychological community. In sandplay we just keep doing what seems irrational or nonprovable. There's no research. So it really has to do with just doing it and knowing there's something there. I remember Jung's response when he was interviewed. He was asked, "Do you believe in God?" And he answered, "I don't believe, I know." It's the difference between believing and having the experience.

MARIA: So what is it that you're experiencing in that silence?

LUCIA: Well, you said "numinous."

MARIA: In the silence we are experiencing the unknown levels of the psyche – the parts of the psyche that are not part of our conscious ego knowing. We are making space in the silence for something to emerge from the unknown and the unconscious that is part of the psyche. And it has its own rhythm and path. We are allowing the silence to emerge and it is allowing the unconscious, unknown parts of us that are numinous and mysterious and shadowy to come forth. We have access to these parts through dreams as well. But, in dreams, you have to use words to translate, which doesn't always hold for the nonverbal, silent part of the dream. And sandplay gives us access to that nonverbal part.

KAY: Exactly.

LUCIA: You know, I think in terms of being a therapist – just thinking about this now – that the client comes in and starts working in the sand, and it's almost like the client gives me an opportunity to once again experience the Self, that numinous place, the nonverbal place. You experience it sometimes when you see a rainbow or hear a child's laughter. There's that moment when everything in the world is perfect and the way it should be – just a moment. I am waiting for the sandplayer to bring us there, so that both of us can be there for that moment, just for that moment. And you and I *know* that it is there, but people can't get to it all the time.

KAY: You have to trust it.

LUCIA: You do have to trust it.

KAY: You have to trust that it's in everybody.

LUCIA: And you have to wait for it! You can't summon it or say, "Okay, now I'm going to do it."

KAY: About this moment – when you experience it together.

MARIA: You were saying you were waiting for that moment. It's so valuable to you.

LUCIA: Yes. At that moment I *know* the reality of the psyche. I *know* that it's there.

KAY: You don't believe in it, you've experienced it.

LUCIA: I've experienced it –

KAY: So you know you can trust it.

LUCIA: And I know that it is there in everyone. And it's like I'm addicted to it. I want it.

KAY: Ah, that's a wonderful thing to say!

LUCIA: I have that same feeling when people say they want to do a tray. There's a little tingle of excitement.

KAY: Mm-hmm, mm-hmm, electricity.

MARIA: There is something unsettling about just focusing on only these numinous, wonderful connections to the psyche, as the only expression of the Self.

LUCIA: I still see the Self, even in the trays that are so disrupted and unsettling.

MARIA: Yeah. Sometimes it's very uncomfortable.

LUCIA: Sometimes that is the experience of that process.

MARIA: The self-guiding something and that's deeper than the ego.

LUCIA: Yes, and it can be quite upsetting.

KAY: And scary.

LUCIA: Very.

MARIA: And that's the beauty and the value of sandplay. Something is being spoken without words.

LUCIA: Yeah.

KAY: It's spoken in symbols.

LUCIA: Yeah, and a symbol is something that we have no words for. We call it a symbol.

MARIA: And yet, the symbol is full of feeling and meaning, and we see the image of that in the sand and it speaks to us.

KAY: On the other hand, there's a universality that we experience in sandplay. It is more universal than language because there are many, many different languages.

MARIA: So there is both the personal and also a universal experience in sandplay.

KAY: Right, but we, as therapists, have to be able to pick up the universal.

MARIA: No sandplayer is going to create the same series as another. All sandplayers develop their own symbol language to get at the universal.

LUCIA: When I work with children, they seem to have a connection with some other space. Sometimes I think they're psychic. They just know things.

KAY: Exactly.

LUCIA: And the older they get and the better their language development becomes, the farther away they get from that knowing place. And it's almost like they illustrate for us what language has done. It pulled us away from nature and Self.

MARIA: There's a book called *The Spell of the Sensuous* [Abram, 1996], and it's about the history of language. Words were originally made from the sounds of nature and animals. This was before there were concepts. Words were connected to sound, like onomatopoeia. So the only words spoken *were* the sounds of humans imitating nature. And just like Stern says about something being lost between mother and baby when words come in, something was also lost when we began to have words with concepts that were disconnected from nature. We lost the rhythm and connection with the seasons, the plants and the animals. Our sounds became further and further from the actual sounds of nature.

LUCIA: Yes. The development of concepts and words actually pulls us away from the central essence of our connection with ourselves, with one another and with nature.

MARIA: According to Lewis, Amini and Lannon, in *A General Theory of Love*, when the limbic system, which is the emotional system of the brain, is developing, the baby's limbic system and the mother's limbic system are in resonance. During early bonding and attachment, there's limbic resonance between mother and baby.

LUCIA: So in doing sandplay we're trying to be there with the sandplayer in this resonance? And – it's not primitive – 'cause it's very evolved –

KAY: Basic.

LUCIA: Okay. All right. So there's another place that we all may experience, either before birth and/or during early development in which we connect profoundly, without words. So, what's silence, then, in our sandplay work? Are we trying to create something – a place –

MARIA: A space.

LUCIA: A space where we can be together –

MARIA: Sandplayer and sandplay therapist.

LUCIA: In that place, that universal place/space. Is that what we're trying to do?

MARIA: Yeah, I think that we're making a space or a place for that nonverbal level of experience to emerge.

KAY: And for the relationship to be deepened.

MARIA: And for the relationship to be deepened and for the relationship to deepen the connection to silence. There is a back and forth resonance.

LUCIA: It is back and forth.

KAY: And that gets us back to the importance of the relationship in silence.

Chapter 6

Silence

Maria Ellen Chiaia

Through meeting in silent relationship, love and hate, despair and joy, boredom and emptiness, loneliness and connection are shared between therapist and sandplayer. These co-transference experiences resonate between and within the sandplayer and the therapist.

In the *Mutus Liber* (McLean, 1991), an alchemical text whose title means "silent book," we see the meeting that occurs in silence as alchemical transformation unfolds. This text was first printed in 1677. Authorship is assigned to a "character" named Altus, which means the high, deep or profound one.

In Plate 4 of that text, the two alchemists enter the field and the work goes on nonverbally. Plate 6 depicts the beginning of the work in the alchemical vessel. In Plate 8 there are angels, messengers of spirit, entering and overseeing the work. The two alchemists are praying silently for inspiration and guidance. One prays passively and the other actively in front of a furnace, the place of transformation. And finally, in Plate 13, one of the last plates, there appears the union of the sun and the moon, the *mysterium coniunctionis*.

The *Mutus Liber* describes an experience in alchemy that is similar to the silent meeting that occurs in sandplay. The images in this text show us the possibilities for transformation that occur when sandplay is engaged in. During relationship in silence, an experience of the *mysterium coniunctionis* is possible. As Jung said, "Every genuine encounter between two human beings must be conceived as a *Mysterium Coniunctionis*. The living mystery of life is always hidden between TWO" (1979, p. 125).

One of the wonderful contributions sandplay brings to our therapeutic work is the value of silence, but even more important is the expression and experience of what happens in that silence. There is the possibility from working in this silent place for a reexperiencing and then a healing of relationship and connection. The sand experience with the therapist and sandplayer engaged in a free and protected place resonates with and to our first human connection, mother and child. And there is a resonance as well to all the subsequent human and nonhuman connections that later occur with animal and plant and in the love of our creator and creation. The mystery of connection and relationship begins in this initial gaze between mother and baby; the miracle of creation begins here for each of us.

While working within the silence of the relationship the sandplayer is touching and feeling the sand and figures that belong to the therapist, while the therapist is engaged in reverie. The feeling and touching that are primary in object relating and in our earliest relationships with our maternal caregivers, and the feeling and touching that happen in sandplay work, are important aspects of silence.

In doing sandplay there can be an emergence and reexperiencing of nonverbal patterns which exist deep in the psychic structures, as well as a finding of new creative patterns within the unconscious. In Jungian psychology we speak of regressive and progressive movements within the psyche, a movement back to these original patterns and a discovery within the unconscious of new patterns and movements. Sandplay shows the path toward deeper layers within ourselves that are potentials needing to be developed. This refers to the progressive movement in the psyche. Jung spoke of this movement when he said that there is a process in the psyche that seeks its own goal.

Let us look at some other writers in the analytic world who describe this process. Balint (1999), in working with the basic fault, speaks about the place of creation. He says that we as analysts have the unique opportunity of observing people while they are absorbed in the area of creation. In order to observe this area of creation we must consider silence not as resistance but as a possible source of information. We must consider what the person is running toward. Balint says that what the person is running toward is a kind of creation, a product of the person's creativity, which deals with the problem which is tormenting the client. However, this creation must occur within the analytic relationship. When working with the basic fault, we need to reestablish a *unio mystica*, the harmonious interpenetrating mix-up. Balint writes:

> The analyst ... must allow his patient to live with him in a sort of harmonious interpenetrating mix ... I am trying to render into words experiences that belong to a period well before or beyond the discovery of words, and largely even before the emergence of objects out of the undisturbed harmony of friendly substances.
>
> (1999, pp. 136–137)

This statement could be related to the creation in sandplay of what we speak of as a free and protected space, a containing space held by the therapist within the silence of relationship. Balint also says that the analyst must not inhibit the unfolding of this process with interpretations. In sandplay we do not interpret at the time the trays are created. We hold the space open, so that the emergence of the sandplayer's material may occur more easily.

There is one other point from Balint that I wish to emphasize about not interpreting. He points out that insight is the result of a correct interpretation. The creation of a proper relationship, however, is required for working on the level of the basic fault and results in feeling. Feeling, Balint explains, is correlated with touching and associated with our most primary object relations, which are created and maintained in a nonverbal interaction between two people. As stated above, when a patient is creating a sandplay, they are witnessed by a therapist who is involved in a reverie about the sandplayer. The sandplayer is touching sand and objects that belong to the therapist. These objects being touched have many different meanings and symbolically have many different relationships to the therapist. Because of all these different meanings and relationships to the therapist, when a patient creates a sandplay we are touched by the touching. Our unconscious responds to the touching and we are filled with images and feelings and associations. But we do not speak, we just note them as we do not want to interfere with this unfolding and the nonverbal relating that is occurring.

Another psychoanalyst, Marion Milner (1969), describes the change of technique needed in working with a woman who had preverbal wounding and was cut off from her creative core. Milner found it necessary to pay attention to the relationship between the articulate and inarticulate, the describable and indescribable. Silence and its essential role in the creation of a safe physical and interpersonal environment are emphasized. Sandplay provides a place where this edge of experience can be held, and then expressed and experienced by the sandplayer and the therapist. As sandplay therapists we experience with the sandplayers the path of the unfolding of their psyche that occurs in and through the silence and the relationship.

Another clinician who has done extensive work with early trauma, Hedges (1994), stresses the importance of the therapist's paying attention, by a different kind of listening, to patterns of self and other affective interactions. Hedges states that we can engage the patient in this way through stories, images, pictures, metaphors and somatic experiences. Sandplay is replete with stories, images, pictures, metaphors and somatic experiences that occur for both the sandplayer creating the tray and therapist observing the tray. Sandplay therapists listen in silence. In working with early trauma and attachment issues, we as sandplay therapists listen and attend to these experiences in the co-transference, for they are an important part of the transformative process in which we are involved.

Sandplay provides a space for the sandplayer to *express*, but more importantly to *experience*, split-off places and for the therapist to experience these places with the sandplayer. In the free and protected space of sandplay therapy I see silence and relationship as the key elements. While sandplay is occurring we do not interpret. A sandplayer needs this space (sitting with a silent therapist) for an inner source of creation (the unconscious) to emerge. The place of creation is where the conscious and unconscious come together in the sandplay therapy.

Finally, Donald Kalsched, in his work on trauma, states:

Great attention must be given to the creation of a safe physical space and a safe interpersonal environment with which dreams and fantasies can emerge and be worked through in a more playful, open-ended fashion than the usual analytic interpretation allows. All forms of the so-called "creative-arts" psychotherapies are extremely helpful toward this end and often these will open up traumatic affect much faster than purely verbal exploration.

(1996, p. 27)

I would like to add that in sandplay not only does traumatic affect emerge, but new patterns and ways of relating to oneself and others also emerge.

I worked with a woman whom I will call Diana, who experienced a great deal of early trauma (Chiaia, 1996). In our silent relationship there was a coldness and disconnection between us that replaced relational warmth and interfered with reverie and playfulness. Sharing the experience of the coldness and disconnection on the one hand and the warmth and container of the analytic space and relationship on the other hand occurred not only in the verbal experiences but also in the spaces between us while she was creating a sandtray.

The experience of the sand work, in the silence of relationship, provided Diana with access not only to the split-off experiences of coldness and disconnection (Figure 6.1) but also to the experience of the mother–child unity and holding. And from that, an experience of wholeness began to unfold (Figure 6.2). She found connection and inner peace while working in the sand. As Dora Kalff said, sandplay:

can establish an inner peace which contains the potential for development of the total personality, including its intellectual and spiritual aspects . . . It is the role of the therapist to perceive these powers and, like the guardian of a precious treasure, protect them in their development.

(1980, p. 30)

Through silence and relationship with sand, water, and miniatures a sandplayer may experience the deepest layers of their psyche, both good and bad, personal and archetypal. With Balint in mind one could say that from the *unio mystica*, the harmonious interpenetrating mix of therapist and sandplayer, a kind of creation may emerge, a product of the sandplayer's creativity which may help sandplayers to deal with the problems that are tormenting them. There is also the possibility of experiencing in the silence of relationship the spiritual, numinous aspects of the psyche, the *mysterium coniunctionis*, or the mystery of meeting, which Jung describes so well.

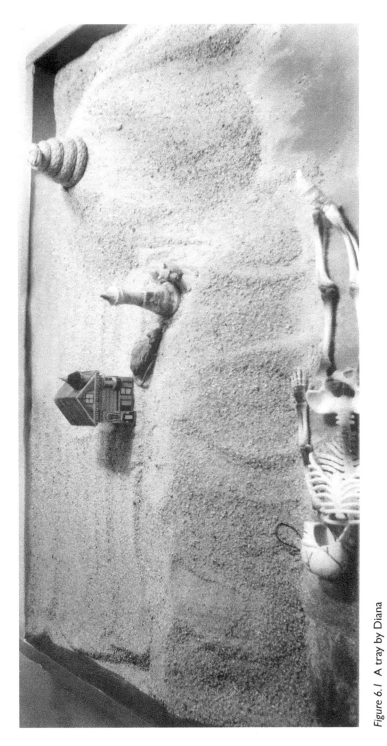

Figure 6.1 A tray by Diana

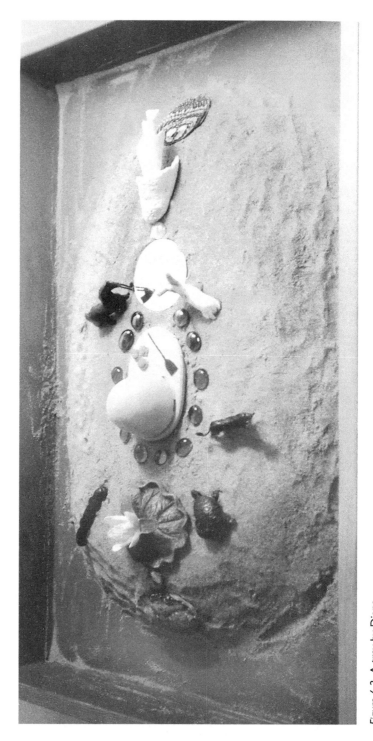

Figure 6.2 A tray by Diana

Chapter 7

Silence

Kay Bradway

Let silence take you to the core of life.
Rumi, 1995

Sandplay therapists appreciate that the silence in sandplay helps clients on their journey to their core. They have observed that the sandplay process allows for easier access to the unconscious than do talk therapies.

Encouraging silence in psychotherapy is unusual. Most psychotherapy is based on verbal dialogue between client and therapist. Sandplay is a nonverbal method not dependent upon words. The instructions given by the therapist to the client usually include the expectation of a nonverbal process. When I was studying with Dora Kalff, she suggested the following instructions: "Look at all the objects on the shelves and when one speaks to you, take it down and put it in the tray and go on as you wish from there." Sometimes sandplayers have had verbal therapy prior to coming for sandplay and expectations to talk are so strong that they do try to make verbal comments about what they are doing or have done. Sandplay therapists have their own way of correcting this misconception. If I knew that a person had previously had therapy, I would say something like, "You may expect that you are supposed to be talking. But you don't have to talk with words. You can just talk with the sand and the figures."

There are several kinds of silence. Karen Signell distinguishes three types: ego silence, which she describes as a conscious silence, "the kind you experience stepping into a library"; natural silence, "the kind you experience walking into the forest"; and deep silence, "a profound state of silence when you enter the deeper layers of the unconscious . . . when you find a more profound and ineffable place within you" (1996, p. 69).

It is Signell's "deep silence" that we experience in sandplay. Usually this is provided by the therapist. But I have three examples in which it was the sandplayer, not the therapist, who provided the silence.

My first example is about a young man whom I had been seeing for several months. A few days before I was to leave on a month's vacation, he came in and went immediately to the sandplay room. Without making any comments, he reached with his fingers through the moist sand to the bottom of the sandtray and made as large an oval as the box permitted. He then proceeded to pat the sand down hard in the oval island, and as he did this, he carefully removed the sand from the edges. He continued patting the sand, adding water occasionally, and stroking and re-stroking the sand into a smoother and smoother *hard* surface. Except for the gentle sound of patting, the room was quiet, silent, resonant with feeling. As he worked I could sense his creating a calmness within himself, and I could also feel myself relaxing. I too felt a calmness being created in me. I felt calmer than I had felt in several days – amid all the pressure of preparing for my trip. The only breaking of the silence was his asking me, about halfway through the hour, what time it was. When I told him that the hour was only halfway up, he gave a sigh of relief and continued.

At the end of the hour he departed with neither of us saying too much, but I felt the depth of what had happened – what had occurred between, and in, both of us. In a small way, in this hour of silence, both of us had experienced a kind of transformation.

Another example, one of someone's creating a *need* for silence, concerns a young woman who came to me for therapy apparently not knowing about sandplay or that I did it. As she walked past the open door to my sandplay room, she wanted to know all about what was in there. In fact, I made it a custom to leave the door to that room open when new people came for their first visit, so that they saw it as they passed by. They often asked me about it, which gave me a chance to tell them about sandplay. They were almost always interested and stimulated. When I explained to this woman what it was all about and said that we might want to use that room sometime in her therapy, she stated in a firm tone that she would never want to do anything like that! We did the usual "get-acquainted" talk for that hour. The next time she came in, she pointed to her throat and whispered hoarsely, "I can't talk." Her laryngitis and not being able to talk necessitated, of course, our going into the non-talk sandplay room. I think it became clear to both of us that her psyche had directed her through her body to the sandplay room. From then on, at almost every visit, she went first of all to the sandplay room and made a sandtray. These sandtrays increasingly contained deep revelations that she wasn't ready to talk about with words. So the sandplay room with the possibility of using images instead of words provided her with the space that apparently was essential for her at that time for eventual healing.

My final sandplay example is about the first client who did sandplay with me. Ida initiated her work in the sandtray by setting up scenes which she thought could illustrate various Jungian theories, and after setting one up she would explain how it related to what she was reading about in books and would ask me questions. Our sessions together were spent in her doing a tray and then our discussing it in detail.

Ida had been referred to me shortly after she had been hospitalized for a psychotic break by a Jungian analyst whom she had been seeing for several years who was moving to another state. I had been doing Jungian analysis for many years but my supervisory hours with Dora Kalff about sandplay had only recently begun. I hadn't yet learned how to handle this kind of situation.

But Ida finally handled it herself. After she had made and talked about nearly 50 sandtrays over a period of a year, she came in one day and put a single figure which represented herself in the center of the tray – all alone. She said nothing about it. This tray marked a turning point in her sandplay process and in the course of her recovery from her illness. From then on we were silent during her making of the scenes and there was no reference to them afterwards. The contrast was amazing!

It would be difficult to overemphasize the contrast between the sand scenes preceding and those following the scene of herself alone. She had left the conscious talking place and the effort of making everything have a rational meaning. She let there be silence, let the psyche take over, and a deep centering and transforming process was activated. This experience deeply moved me. When I shared this experience by letter with Dora Kalff, she replied in part: "This proves what I say that a silent understanding constellates the synchronistic moment from where the next step evolves" (Bradway and McCoard, 1997, p. 130).

I want to end by sharing a moving account about silence by someone who was not a sandplayer or a client, but a concert pianist. At the time that this musician was scheduled to play a Bartók composition in a concert, he learned that Bartók himself was going to be in the audience. He was both frightened and elated. He played his very best. After the performance, Bartók came up to him and said, "You played the notes very well. Do not forget to play the silences – as well."

Chapter 8

Silence

Lucia Chambers

Creative ideas took shape in the inner and outer stillness.
(Jaffe, 1972, p. 133)

It might be helpful to look at the definition of silence in order to be able to understand why sandplay considers it so important. Webster defines silence as "the absence of any sound or noise" (Barnhart, 1947). Already we are in difficulty because as long as there is a human consciousness, there is sound, a noise of some kind. Even floating in an immersion tank, where silence was sought in the 1960s, there was sound. As the noises of the external world were blocked out, the internal sounds became very audible. The pulse drummed in the inner channel of the ear. The pounding of the heart seemed as if it might cause ripples in the water. The whish of the blood in the arteries was like the waves of the ocean gently breaking on the sands. The inner sounds that had been present all the time, but not heard, now could claim our attention. So perhaps we need to clarify what sound or noise is absent when we are in a silent state. Again, Webster defines what it is to be silent: "making no sound; quiet; still; refraining from speech; speechless; mute" (Barnhart, 1947).

There has been an awareness, down through the centuries, that a person's individual experience of living can be altered simply by being in it without words. This "altered state" seems to open doors to a deeper level of wisdom and inspiration that causes the consciousness to assume a totally different perspective on life, its meaning and intention, and the individual's place within it. So when groups of people come together seeking ways to precipitate this altering experience, the form created is frequently that of silence.

There is a villa, north of Pompeii, which is thought to have been built between 31 BC and AD 14. The walls of the front room are covered with brilliant frescoes depicting, symbolically, in ten scenes, the Orphic ritual of initiation for aristocratic women of that time. The third scene is described by Linda Fierz-David, a docent at the Jung Institute in Zurich: "The tender chirping tone of the old stringed instrument, which perhaps most nearly resembles a bird song. This tender tone, the alluring voice that sounds up from the unconscious and announces the Self, can only be heard *when the human being does not speak"* (1988, p. 60). This secret, sacred ritual had silence as an essential component for deepening the mystery, knowing that only when the human voice is quiet can the space be open for the speaking of another voice.

About AD 800, Saint Benedict formulated the 72 Rules that facilitate a contemplative life devoted to a quest for God. Silence is for me a prerequisite for a conversation with God. Sometimes the human voice can overwhelm the whispers of the soul. The Benedictines, the Trappists, the Carmelites, the Poor Clares all knew that words, even those eloquent in praise and adulation, filled the ear and heart so that a deeper message would be missed.

In Oliver Cromwell's England, in the early 1650s, there was a deep disillusionment with the functioning of the Christian Church. The leaders of the Church were much interested in politics and used the Holy Book and the sacraments to communicate God's wishes to man. Small groups of men and women began to gather in their homes, intent upon going beyond words about God to a personal experience of the Mystery. Silence was the primary ingredient in that experience. Rufus Jones, writing about the early history of the Quakers, records,

> The early Friends made the discovery that silence is one of the best preparations for communion [with God] and for the reception of inspiration and guidance. Silence itself, of course, has no magic. It may be just sheer emptiness, absence of words or noise or music. It may be an occasion for slumber, or it may be a dead form. But it may be an intensified pause, a vitalized hush, a creative quiet, an actual moment of mutual and reciprocal correspondence with God.
>
> (1937, par. 244)

Inspiration and guidance, communion with God, the voice of the Self rising from the unconscious, are all different ways of explaining the nonverbal, silent presence of the sandplay therapist when someone is creating a picture in the sand. In that space, free from the confining definitions of the human voice, the path is open for a message from the deepest layer of the unconscious.

The collective unconscious contains all patterns ever experienced by humankind. It is from this deep and vast psychological space that energies rise up and help one choose from the little figures on the shelves. These figures are only forms that represent those energies. If they are labeled or identified, or words imposed upon them, the message to be delivered is immediately closed in and restricted. Words wound these archetypal energies because words are totally unable to express the unlimited potential for creation that lies in the depths – the Self, God. That immenseness can only be contained in the nonverbal experience of the client, shared by the therapist, as it is symbolically expressed in a free and protected space. Poets can use words in the richest and most exquisite way to attempt to capture the essence in words, but even they can't quite do it. Rumi says,

> This is how it always is
> when I finish a poem.
> A great silence overcomes me,
> and I wonder why I ever thought
> to use language.
>
> 1995, p. 20

Our relationship to silence is decidedly ambivalent. We have known since the beginning of conscious time that silence, or being without words, gives us a better opportunity to receive a message from that place beyond our present understanding. We meditate and pray in silence. We have a moment of silence when we honor the memory of a tragedy. We whisper in places that have a profound presence: in cathedrals, at funerals, and in a forest of ancient redwoods. We pay substantial fees for silent retreats. And at the same time, we bombard ourselves with television in banks, in restrooms, in store windows and in church vestibules. We have stereo systems operating in places of entertainment and in cars that have a volume capable of permanently damaging the ears of our children. We have "call waiting," which assures us that we will not miss the opportunity to talk with yet another person.

Again we turn to Webster for assistance. "Ambivalence: the coexistence of opposite and conflicting feelings about the same person or object" (Barnhart, 1947). The silence that holds the sought-for wisdom holds not only the ecstatic revelations experienced by the mystics, but also dark pain and surrender. The living energy, the Self, which has the ability to move us into a new space and a new awareness of life, requires us first to sacrifice that which we have always been. Jung said, "Creation is as much destruction as construction" (1969b, par. 245). According to the symbolic thinking of the alchemists, the identity that has been created by the ego must be smashed, burned and dismembered before the sublime gold will emerge. Similarly, sand scenes can show conflict, chaos, death and destruction for many weeks or months before there is a picture with some harmony and peace. Death comes before birth. The ego, with its carefully constructed and restrictive defenses, must surrender to the greater vision of the Self. The sandplay therapist watches as these opposing forces confront each other in the sand. Only then can the transcendent function lift consciousness to another level. The edges of the sand box and the experienced psyche of the therapist hold and contain this battle to the death, allowing it to play out in that protected space rather than in the dangerous open space of everyday life. Therapists sit in that place of no words, hold and wait, turning themselves over to the deeper wisdom of the process.

> Silence is the language of God;
> It is also the language of the heart.
>   Dag Hammarskjöld

Part III

Child

Chapter 9

Child trialogue

LUCIA: One of the things that I think is wonderful about the history of sand-play is that before Dora Kalff and sandplay, as I understand it, Jungian psychology was applicable only to adults. And the story that I heard – and I love these stories because nobody can say they're not true – is that Jung – Carl and Emma – conferred with Dora when she finished her course of education and said, "You are so gifted with children. Can Jungian psychology apply also to children?" She then went to the Lowenfeld Clinic in London and started to observe children. As she observed their play, she found that the individuation process could be seen in the sand. This is the story I heard. No?

KAY: The story I love is that Jung's grandchildren used to go over to play with Dora's children. And when they went back home, they seemed so much better. They seemed healthier and happier. So Jung asked Dora, "What do you do?" And she said, "We just play." Jung was attracted by this and realized that Dora had a special gift with children. So he encouraged her when she said she wanted to go to Margaret Lowenfeld and study.

LUCIA: So Dora wanted to go?

KAY: Yes, I think so and she checked with Jung and he said, "Oh, yes. That would be a good idea." So Dora went to London to study with Lowenfeld who had already created her World Technique using the sandtray and miniature figures.

LUCIA: Yes.

KAY: After Dora started to include the World Technique in her play therapy with children, she realized it didn't depend upon the sandtray's telling the therapist about the child. It was the experience of the child in using the sandtray and the relationship with the therapist that did it.

MARIA: Kay, can you say more about that last part?

KAY: Well, Lowenfeld tried to avoid transference to any one particular therapist. I understand that she had different therapists see the same children so the transference would be to the building, not to a therapist.

LUCIA: Or the therapist's green apron.

KAY: When I studied with John Hood-Williams, who was a student of Margaret Lowenfeld, he thought that the sandtray showed the therapist what was going on in the child's mind and feelings and the therapist would use it that way. Dora realized that it was the experience of playing in the sand, in what she called the free and protected space provided by an empathic therapist, that did it. I think that was her great contribution.

LUCIA: Uh-huh.

KAY: And I think it has been shown that night dreaming, even if the dreams are not recalled, is conducive to psychological health.

MARIA: Was Lowenfeld against interpretation?

KAY: No.

MARIA: She was just against the transference?

KAY: Yes.

MARIA: So, then, Dora Kalff emphasized the actual process and the transference rather than the interpretation?

KAY: That's the thing. I always explain it by saying it's experience, not explanation, that heals.

LUCIA: Not even the therapist's seeing it and understanding it, but the experience of doing the sandplay itself that is healing.

KAY: Yes, that is the individuation process. But there has to be the empathic therapist providing the space, the tray and the miniature collection.

MARIA: It is the playing in the sand with the therapist present that is the healing.

KAY: It is the process that is healing. It doesn't have to be explained. And this is different from many other depth therapies.

LUCIA: It's so hard for us to believe that there is an actual, living energy that is working in the moment. It's almost impossible for people to get it – to believe that that's true. So what children need, then, is the opportunity for the experience of a free and protected space for this energy to work. It is a natural thing for children to play. They do it intuitively, do they not?

KAY: I don't think the use of play as therapy with children was accepted until the time that Child Guidance Clinics were started in the late 1930s or early 1940s. The idea of a therapist's playing with a child, rather than just asking them questions or trying to analyze their dreams or sometimes their drawings, was new. I think this was independent of Jungian or Kalffian therapy. Jung didn't provide for child therapy in his work. Michael Fordham, of course, came along and focused his work on children, and did play with them. But he never really approved of sandplay therapy. Erich Neumann proposed important theories about child development that Dora later verified in her work with children. But Neumann did not actually do any therapy with children. I think it was in Child Guidance Clinics that play therapy really took off.

LUCIA: And even the name of those child clinics was interesting: Guidance? It insinuates that the adult is there to guide the child rather than the psyche of the child being there to guide the adult therapist. There has been a monumental shift in our belief system on our perspectives of children. I never like to hear people say, "Oh, that child is acting out" – as something bad.

KAY: I don't either. It's awful.

LUCIA: And if – if we could shift our perspective and say, "All right. This child is doing – being – the way they are because of what is happening inside and the child is trying to shift –"

KAY: Or cope. They're coping. And the coping process is the healing process.

LUCIA: So the acting out then, essentially, is a positive thing that we can – we need to pay attention to.

KAY: We need to give a free and protected space for it, unless, of course, it puts someone in physical danger.

LUCIA: There needs to be a space for what is being acted out to express itself. Instead, we give them Ritalin. And I wonder, too, about the popularity of the ADD diagnosis. What are those children trying to say who are overactive, uncooperative and have a low attention span? What are they doing?

KAY: They're trying to do something to help themselves. They are calling out for understanding. But they are given something like Ritalin to try and stop their call.

LUCIA: So what is trying to be expressed gets repressed. And then we have a situation like Columbine – when it comes out, when they're big enough to *really* act out. Oh! That distresses me.

KAY: The students in that situation had not had a free and protected space earlier to act out in a small way, so now they were acting out in a big way and it was tragic.

LUCIA: So there is this intuitive place in the child that knows what they need to do to grow and develop.

KAY: The other thing that I think is interesting is that the child knows how they are perceived and this makes a difference.

LUCIA: What do you mean?

KAY: Well, when the teacher, or parent, perceives the child as a nuisance or as a problem, then the child becomes more like that. I think you tend to become how you are perceived.

LUCIA: Out of the need to belong and be accepted?

KAY: Then being a nuisance identifies you in some way. At least you are an individual. And you take on how others perceive you and you are that way.

MARIA: In what you are describing, there are not many possibilities for the child. There is a narrowness of perception and identification, and also a squishing inside the child of daydreaming and play, both of which are connected to the imagination. There is not much room to take on different roles and identities. What I'm finding in my practice is that younger and younger children are disconnected from the imagination.

LUCIA: From the natural.

MARIA: From the natural creative process.

LUCIA: Right.

MARIA: There is very little time and space for the child to daydream or imagine. They go from one activity to the next. And there is pressure to be good at scholastics as well as all the many after-school activities such as music, art, swimming, gymnastics, sports, and so forth.

LUCIA: And dance.

MARIA: There's no room for a child to just sit quietly and daydream or fantasize or make up stories.

LUCIA: That's right. Or there is not much consideration for individual pacing. It may not be the time for all seven-year-old boys to take Aikido. We're putting our children in boxes.

MARIA: I find that some children come into my office and have no response to the collection. There is not an immediate relationship with the collection and the room as being numinous or magical.

LUCIA: Is that right?

KAY: That's horrible.

MARIA: I was used to getting that response from preteens or teenagers, but this is happening with kids who are eight and ten years old.

LUCIA: Doesn't the sand pull them?

MARIA: No, they have little inner ability to imagine. One little girl looked at the sand collection and said, "Well, I don't know what to make." The figures or the sand did not draw her in. I had to help her make the connection to her inner experience. I knew she loved animals so I said something like, "Well, let's make something with animals."

LUCIA: So what you're doing, then, is helping her rediscover her Self, her inner Self.

KAY: With freedom and protection of the space.

MARIA: Also, I am helping her to find the connection to her inner world through her imagination and her ability to play.

LUCIA: I have had similar experiences with children and I have found that they can play with the dollhouse and they can play games.

MARIA: The lack of imagination is connected with attachment difficulties.

LUCIA: "Attachment disorders," a lot of us realize – what a big problem that is now. We're attaching to computers. What the disorder is, or what is out of kilter, is the ability to attach, or connect, or be in relationship to the natural Self. "Attachment disorder" usually means you don't attach to a person. You don't like mommy, or you can't accept another person as important. The reason that the child can't do that is because they, themselves, are not connected with their inner Self.

MARIA: And that connection with the inner Self was not established and needed to be established in the relationship with the mother.

LUCIA: Things are changing. About five or six years ago when a parent called in to bring their child into therapy and the child sometimes didn't want to come, I would say, "Well, bribe them. Take them to McDonald's or give them cookies or whatever." And then, when they got into my office, in the room with my sand collection, they wanted to come back. Every single child, when they saw the sand and the little figures, wanted to come back. Now are you saying that –

KAY: Has changed?

MARIA: There's somewhat of a change – yes.

LUCIA: Ah! That is very frightening.

MARIA: There are still the children that can and *do* get right in the sand but I'm seeing more children that aren't making that connection.

LUCIA: That is frightening. Some people say that the computer games for children are creative. Do you think? So the time when the child would – might – need to be daydreaming –

KAY: Or making up their games.

LUCIA: Instead, they're in a chair in front of something that's already structured and all they have to do is push a button. They don't have to create a character. They don't have to – what?

KAY: Imagine.

MARIA: There's also all the video and visual stimulation as well. It doesn't allow for that ability to imagine either. Unlike reading. When you're reading something, you have to imagine what that looks like.

KAY: That's why reading *Harry Potter* is better than seeing it.

LUCIA: When the child is free to be whoever and wherever they need to be, at that particular moment in time, that is what Dora's free space is all about, isn't it?

KAY: It's uncommon to have both freedom and protection. But they should have times when they have both.

LUCIA: And where else in their life can they do that?

KAY: Unless they've had a very good mother. I've been in houses of the same age child where one house is just a mess, and it's fine. The child is getting along great. And another house where everything is neat and the child is apparently unhappy. And I know the priorities are wrong. Neatness of house is more important than happiness of child.

LUCIA: The longer we talk about it, the more scared I get.

KAY: Mm-hmm. Yeah, I think this is very good.

LUCIA: So as therapists now, we are realizing that children are being –

KAY: Deprived.

LUCIA: Deprived, banished, and damaged, and the natural creative aspect of the child's Self is being shut down.

KAY: Thwarted.

MARIA: And not nurtured.

LUCIA: Thwarted and not nurtured. What are we as therapists going to do?

MARIA: As therapists we can only do so much. Certainly, we need to expand on our ideas of what the free and protected space means. The free and protected space includes –

KAY: Attachment to the therapist.

MARIA: Attachment to the therapist, attachment to the space –

KAY: Or whatever it takes, before they get to the sand.

MARIA: As therapists, we are having to take steps to get them there rather than assuming the child is going to come in and be swept up by the sand collection.

LUCIA: It won't – it doesn't work that way.

KAY: Well, that's interesting because that's what modern-day, coming-to-be therapists would feel. They would feel thwarted and discouraged if a child came into their sandplay room and didn't connect with the sand. Knowing that this is what is happening encourages therapists to continue even though they feel discouraged.

LUCIA: That's right. That's right.

MARIA: But it is very sad to see this disconnection in a child when the child comes into the sandplay room. It's very sad.

LUCIA: How do you work with this, Maria?

MARIA: Well, I try to connect with the child around the things that matter to them. I find out what those things are that matter.

LUCIA: But what if they say, "Captain Something," a game, or something on TV or on a computer? Where do you go with that?

MARIA: Well, I need to find out about the game. I need to know what they are attracted to in the game. Then I'll talk with them about that. I'll try to make some connection for them about what matters and has meaning for them.

KAY: The very fact you're trying to make that connection is marvelously healing to the child. They may not get that kind of attention very often.

MARIA: I recall a little girl who loved dogs. So she brought her dog to our sessions and I brought mine, and we played with the dogs in the yard. Slowly we began to make a connection through the dogs.

KAY: Mm-hmm. Good.

LUCIA: Something I have found useful, particularly with teenagers, is ritual. For instance, rocks and crystals really appeal to them. With a very angry young man, we talked about how the earth and the rocks absorb water, and how the earth and the rocks absorb whatever falls to the earth. I asked him, "What if you carried a rock in your pocket? And when you feel this anger, how about putting your hand on the rock and letting the anger go into the rock and stay in the rock?" This guy wore black leathers, spiked hair and chains: he was a scary-looking guy, 16 years old. He loved it! And every time he brought back this rock, he said, "Okay. Now we need to drain this rock."

KAY: That's wonderful!

LUCIA: So we drained it. And then he put it back in his pocket.

MARIA: Mm-hmm. I love that.

LUCIA: So the ancient rituals hold the sacred or the connection with nature. The Native Americans know it and we know it, too, on a deeper level. And a little girl loved crystals, " 'cause they're pretty." And then I read with her that rose quartz increases confidence and gives comfort. She loved that! And then we made a little piece of jewelry. We used a little ritual to lead the way back to the real Self. Sometimes in the beginning, if they don't like the toys, they may still like the natural things: rocks and –

KAY: Seeds and acorns.

LUCIA: That's right. All children love the little natural things or objects belonging to ancient cultures native to different regions of the world.

MARIA: All this helps the children to connect with the inner and outer through –

KAY: Nature or the nonhuman.

LUCIA: You remember Dora said in her video that one of the problems is that we're losing connection with the instinctual Self? And the instinctual Self is the part that heals and develops and individuates. To go back to the instinctual, perhaps, with animals –

MARIA: Or through natural objects, and then making a connection through a ritual that works for a particular child so that they begin to imagine numinosity in the outer world, in the figures or in nature.

KAY: They experience something they may never have experienced before.

MARIA: And then there is an inner and outer connection –

KAY: That is healing and the basis of individuation.

MARIA: What we're having to do now is take more steps to get them into the sand, because the TV, the videos, and the computers compete with the figures.

LUCIA: They do. We need to learn a little bit more about how to draw them in.

KAY: I think we can do this through the relationship. We can do things that make children feel appreciated, understood, cherished. Just paying attention to what they say – listening. Or letting them know we enjoy being with them. Or reinforcing their feeling good about themselves. I used to tell mothers two things to do: "When your child has accomplished something that they feel good about, say something like 'You must feel good about yourself for doing that.' " It's not complimenting or saying how you feel about it, but it's validating their own good feelings about themselves that I think is important. And secondly, I would tell mothers, "Let them know when you feel joy in being with them."

LUCIA: And as therapists we are joyful with them and we can let them know.

KAY: Yeah, joyful. The mothers seemed to be surprised at this. But it worked and their relationship with their child improved. And I think as therapists we can and do naturally use these two techniques. This is quite different from using images in the sandtray, but I think this is another part of it. This is the relationship part of the therapy.

MARIA: That's a very important piece, Kay. In this day and age, the parents are so busy they may not remember or know, or take the time for that. Or sometimes they can't find the joy in themselves, so then we are left providing this joy. It is important then for us to reflect our joy upon seeing the child or reflect to the child when the child feels good about itself.

KAY: Yes, that's what I mean. And as therapists, we can do it.

MARIA: So that is part of the free and protected space. With most children, I smile when I see them.

KAY: Yeah. Well, you probably do enjoy it.

MARIA: It is so important to bring this joy and pleasure into the child's life, this joy and pleasure to see them. So the child may feel lovely.

LUCIA: Isn't that what we do with the creation of sand pictures? We acknowledge them and may say, "You must be feeling good about what you've done."

MARIA: Isn't that beautiful – lovely.

LUCIA: Isn't that wonderful. Those are the two things that we do.

KAY: Yeah. We are appreciating what they're doing, even though there may be chaos in the tray.

MARIA: We are not judging the sandtray; we are appreciating the playing, the doing, the creating of the sandtray and how they may feel about it.

LUCIA: So we're taking care of the inner child all the time. There's a poem by Mary Richards, which I can't quote, but it says something like: "In the face of every grown man I can see the child" [Richards, 1962] The inner child is there and needs the same recognition, approval, love and acknowledgment as a child. I can't find too much difference, sometimes, in seeing adults, if I talk to that inner child.

KAY: But of course, with children, the whole room is part of the therapy. With adults, usually, unless you're doing sandplay therapy, you are just with them.

LUCIA: That's right. That's the difference.

MARIA: I'd like to spend the last bit of time talking about the child in the adult and that ability of the adult to come in and play. It is difficult for some people to connect to the sandplay or the collection, or to that playful, child-like or creative part of themselves.

KAY: Especially men.

LUCIA: Well, we've already done it to them, you see. By the time they're adults, the child is hiding. And that's really sad.

MARIA: So how do we get them into the sandplay?

KAY: When one therapist observed that more women used sandplay than men did, I noted that all the men I was seeing at that time made some use of sandplay. And the very using of it – even the first time – had been healing. It was such a break for the men to do something so different. Men have lost this ability to play more than women have.

LUCIA: Of course they have! They're out there competing with everybody. And it doesn't matter that they need to have their own pace and time to just sit back. The men think they'd better not sit back. We all have to grow up and function in an adult world, but how can we keep the child alive?

MARIA: And how can we keep the imaginal alive?

LUCIA: That's what a child is, a child is playful.

MARIA: Playing is part of the human life at all stages. The ability to play and imagine and be creative is our birthright. And children as well as adults are being denied their birthright. It takes its toll on the whole society.

LUCIA: You bet!

MARIA: People actually fare better – intellectually – if they have their creativity nurtured.

LUCIA: Nurtured – from the beginning.

KAY: And, if they haven't had it nurtured from the beginning, then providing a creative, playful space for both children and adults is essential.

LUCIA: When the adults haven't had the encouragement in the beginning, we get the phenomenon of burnout. They use up the few resources they have stored up and they have little ability to create and imagine what else could come. There's nothing beyond.

MARIA: But we, as sandplay therapists, try to make a space for them.

LUCIA: We try. That's it.

MARIA: Well, I like that we call ourselves sandplay therapists, because we emphasize the play rather than the making of a sandtray. The making of a sandtray is not the purpose of it. The purpose of it is to play.

KAY: Yes, to play. I've heard it said that more male therapists would take up sandplay therapy if it were called something else – something that didn't use the word "play."

LUCIA: To eliminate "play" is to eliminate the whole understanding of sandplay therapy.

KAY: The whole point.

MARIA: The idea that playing is therapy is a very important idea.

Chapter 10

Child

Maria Ellen Chiaia

According to Winnicott, "playing is immensely exciting ... a kind of magic that arises in intimacy, in a relationship that is reliable ... motivated by the mother's love or her love/hate" (1986, p. 47). He goes on to say that when a child cannot play this is a major symptom that must be attended to. Most children have a magical experience of the sandplay collection. However, there are some children who do not have this experience. This may be due to problems of attachment and/or overstimulation due to television, video and computer activities as well as from just too many scheduled activities.

In working with these children, attending to the creation of a free and protected space through our relationship to the child is essential. Attending to and working in the co-transference is needed. Also, it is important to see the child in a positive light even if the child is presenting with very difficult behaviors and symptoms. I would go so far as to say we have to love the child, seeing something good and appreciating them each time we see them. Over time, children respond to our empathic caring, begin to learn about themselves through our experience of them and eventually begin to open up. Slowly the child may risk sharing inner feelings, dreams and thoughts, allowing the therapist to engage with these parts of themselves. An imaginal play begins and is nurtured by the therapist. The therapist must treat this emerging play as a fragile little seedling that needs protection and care.

As the seedling is fed and watered, it grows; the imaginal play expands from this sharing. Eventually the imaginal play includes some of the sandplay toys and leads to the creation of a sand picture. Sometimes adults have a child inside who has never played or has forgotten how to play, and we engage the adult in the same way so that playing may become possible.

Play occurs in an in-between space, between inner and outer experience (Winnicott, 1986, p. 41). When the therapist who is outside empathizes and takes interest in a child's inner world (even before the creation of a sand picture), an inner and outer, verbal and nonverbal, dialogue begins. This dialogue develops into communicative play and meaning is created between therapist and child. We assist children in creating stories about their inner experiences as these stories eventually flower into playing and the creation of a sand picture. Imaginative play begins to flourish.

In sandplay, in the creation of a sand picture, we may give birth to a new part of ourselves or this part of ourselves may be experienced for the first time with another. It may appear as a birth and relate to the archetypal or divine child. The child archetype is an aspect of individuation. In individuation the symbol of the child represents the figure that synthesizes the conscious and unconscious elements of the personality; it unites the opposites and makes whole.

In children's and in adults' sandtrays we may find abandoned, lonely, hurt, exposed children – motifs we find in myths about child heroes or child gods. This refers to the personal difficulties a child or adult has suffered as well as difficulties faced in the individuation. Jung writes:

> Nothing in all the world welcomes this new birth, although it is the most precious fruit of Mother Nature herself, the most pregnant with the future, signifying a higher state of realization. That is why Nature, the world of instincts, takes the "child" under its wing: it is nourished or protected by animals.
>
> (Jung and Kerenyi, 1973, p. 87)

When animals and their babies, or animals protecting human babies, appear in a sandtray, we are warmed and feel hopeful, because the feeling of wholeness and containment in the Self is being experienced. This new Self has emerged and it is being protected.

In children we feel potential and possibility, as they are at the beginning of life. The symbol of the child holds this same potential and possibility. But Jung takes this idea of beginning and expands it to include the end. He states that the symbol of the child is:

> both the beginning and end . . . Psychologically speaking, this means that the "child" symbolizes the pre-conscious and post-conscious essence of man. His pre-conscious essence is the unconscious state of earliest childhood; his post-conscious essence is an anticipation by analogy of life after death. In this idea the all-embracing nature of psychic wholeness is expressed . . . The "child" is all that is abandoned and exposed and at the same time divinely powerful; the insignificant, dubious beginning, and the triumphal end. The "eternal child" in man is an indescribable experience, an incongruity, a handicap, and a divine prerogative; an imponderable that determines the ultimate worth or worthlessness of a personality.
>
> (Jung and Kerenyi, 1973, pp. 97–98)

Jung of course is speaking not of the human child but of the archetype of the eternal, divine child.

Sandplay provides the human child or the child within the adult with the opportunity to play. And through playing, as inner and outer, conscious and unconscious meet, the sandplayer may experience the personal child from infancy and childhood and/or the archetypal divine child, the Self. We may experience all that is abandoned and neglected and/or all that is divinely powerful. Whatever we encounter will engage the child and play, as well as engaging the archetype of child. And there will be the opportunity to touch and experience the "eternal child," an experience that cannot be described in words but only in images. Jung described the "eternal child" in man as an "indescribable experience" (1973, p. 98). Sandplay, by engaging our conscious and unconscious through play, may enable us to have this indescribable experience.

Chapter 11

Child

Kay Bradway

Two approaches to therapy with children have emerged within the Jungian framework. Jung left no guidelines, since he and his early followers adhered to the idea that children's problems depended largely on the projections of their parents' shadows upon them. Children were cured by curing their parents. About the same time that Michael Fordham was developing his child therapy based on some of the work of the Freudian Melanie Klein, Dora Kalff was developing sandplay therapy referring to some of the theories of the Jungian Erich Neumann.

Fordham's and Kalff's approaches to child therapy are generally recognized as being divergent from one another, with Fordham focusing on the developmental with interpretation and Kalff focusing on imaging in sandplay with avoidance of interpretation. Tom Kirsch notes: "In San Francisco, as in other centers of the world, the two approaches diverged more than they complemented each other" (2000, p. 88).

To make a comparison of the two approaches, Brian Feldman and I, both teaching at the C.G. Jung Institute of San Francisco, compared the therapy processes of two children whom we had seen in analysis, Brian's using Fordham's developmental approach with a seven-year-old boy and mine using sandplay with a nine-year-old girl. As we looked at the course of the therapy with the two children, we found a number of common aspects despite marked differences in the two children and the nature and etiology of their problems. Underlying both was the power of self-healing. Given freedom to do what they wanted in a safe place provided by an empathic therapist, these children themselves directed the therapy.

Appreciating the significance of our findings, Brian and I co-authored the article "Child analysis using Kalff and Fordham" (Bradway and Feldman, 2002). What follows is edited versions of our two summaries of our therapies with the two children, our list of common aspects of the therapies, and our concluding remarks.

Brian's summary of Bobby

Developmental history indicated that Bobby was good-natured as a young infant. At ten months, difficulties with swallowing followed by several surgeries ended up in a condition that was properly labeled psychotic. When I first saw him, he would not talk directly to me. Play included the dismantling of objects, taking apart of pencils and pens, cutting small dolls into pieces. The playroom was put into a state of disarray.

Contact was eventually made through Bobby's use of a stuffed dog. He said that the dog wanted to kill me. Gradually the dog began to relate to me more and more. Initially, Bobby said the dog hated nipples and wanted to tear my "wee-wee" (penis) off. Later, the dog began to be punished for hating me. Gradually Bobby started to tell me his dreams.

Bobby then began to approach me more directly, but often in an aggressive manner. He attempted to place objects inside my clothing, in particular a small stuffed animal, a mouse he named "Miss Squeak," who became a transitional object mediating between Bobby and me. Gradually themes were enacted with the use of this stuffed animal. At times Bobby wanted Squeak inside me so I could hold her safely. Other times, she was associated with an aggressive baby who wanted to tear out my insides. Squeak would want to eat me in order to control me. Bobby began to call me "Dr Weirdman" or "Dr Madman." It appeared he was attempting to project the psychotic part of his personality into me so I could help him digest his unmetabolized and uncontained aggression and rage. He tried to control my every move in the sessions. At times he tried to attack my penis and anus. As he attacked me, I also became aware of angry feelings in myself. The depth of feeling and fantasy he evoked made me aware of how much he needed to communicate his rage and desperation and how he needed to utilize my capacity for thought and imagination to help him experience containment and safety.

Prior to the summer break, Bobby asked to take a turtle puppet home so he would have some remembrance of me in the absence.

Later, after marked ambivalence that emerged in the transference, Bobby surprisingly said to me, "You're a good person because you help me think about my problems."

Experiences of integration for Bobby involved moments of feeling inwardly calm, alive, and loving. As therapy progressed, more progress was noted by his caregivers in his relationship to the external world and in his relationships at home and at school. There was more capacity for concentration and learning, and interpersonal relationships became less strained by anxiety and aggression.

Kay's summary of Kathy

Kathy was nine years old and having increasing difficulties in school when she was referred to me for sandplay therapy. A diagnostic evaluation read in part, "Serious emotional problems related to low self-esteem and inability to assert herself in interpersonal relationships. At least average intelligence, but poor written language and poor visual–motor coordination, supporting a diagnosis of dyslexia." Her father, who had been very critical of her inabilities in school, often accusing her of "not trying," had died four months previously.

Kathy avoided verbal interchanges with me but took readily to sandplay. In her initial tray and several later trays she placed fences around animals, especially after any show of anger or even assertiveness, reflecting her need to find ways of controlling expressions of her anger. For example, after a tray in which Kathy had us shoot toy cannons at each other, and after a tray portraying a cannon shooting at a mother bawling out her daughter, she made trays at the next sessions with fenced-in animals. Gradually she was able to make trays with animals outside of fences.

Many of Kathy's trays showed a concern about the differences between boys and girls, bad and good, children and grownups, which gradually gave way to a greater union of these. For example: At first, all boys in the trays were described as bad and all girls as good; later, there were both good boys and bad girls. Initially, gardens were separated from school; later, they were combined. At first, children were in a school and grownups outside; later, grownups were put into a school. Finally, she made a tray that portrayed a "city for everyone," with boys and girls, children and grownups, black children, Native Americans, Japanese.

Kathy asserted herself by asking me to put together some play items. She mocked me when I had trouble. Then when I succeeded, she gloated, "I told you you could do it."

There was an instance when Kathy wanted to take objects out of a closet. I felt it necessary to thwart her wishes since the closet was not mine. We had a controversy about this. I felt truly anxious and angry. I finally became more lenient and withdrew my strict prohibition. She experienced "winning."

When vacation caused a separation, Kathy brought me a pencil sharpener the last day before her vacation. She also wrote "Love" on the blackboard.

In her final sandplay scene Kathy had us make a castle out of sand together and said a princess lived in the castle and explained, "Her father keeps her there." I asked if he was mean to her, and she replied, "No. He protects her." She then had us both shoot at the castle together, saying that the princess went to the bottom of the castle while the battle was going on, where she was able to protect herself. In looking for a lost bullet, Kathy destroyed the whole thing. I think this marked the freeing of herself from the negative father complex, with an appreciation of the positive masculine and its use by the ego. She seemed to have fully experienced both the negative side of the otherwise good feminine and the positive side of otherwise bad masculine.

In an early scene Kathy depicted a stream and said it had poison in it. In her final scene she depicted a stream and said, "It goes under a bridge and comes out pure." In her last session in the sandplay room Kathy drew on the blackboard a boy and a girl going to a party.

I saw Kathy once a month in my office for the next six months, at which time her school work and interpersonal relationships had shown steady improvement. Therapy was terminated by mutual consent. Later communication from her mother indicated a happier child and included report cards showing all good grades.

Common aspects

Brian and I found several common aspects in the therapies of the two children despite the gender difference, age difference (Bobby seven; Kathy nine), the difference in apparent age at which their development suffered disruption (Bobby about ten months, Kathy about six years), and the nature of the disruption (Bobby, lack of proper containment, the mother level: loved for being; Kathy, lack of appropriate response to her achievement, the father level: loved for doing).

Common aspects we found in the two therapies were as follows.

1 Both children initially avoided all verbal communication.
2 Both communicated through toys.
3 Both were in control of the play and the toys (dog; miniatures).
4 Both were concerned with "good" and "bad."
5 Both used therapy to help with fear of uncontrolled anger.
6 Both showed negative feelings toward the therapist through the use of "toys." Bobby said the dog wanted to kill Brian. Kathy had Kay and her shoot toy cannons at each other.
7 Both put therapist in a position in which the child could experience being the authority. (Brian: "He tried to control my every move." Kay: "She had me put together items and mocked me when I had trouble.")
8 Both therapists became aware of angry feelings in themselves.
9 Both children, on the day before a separation from therapist, provided for a passing of a concrete object between therapist and child that was appropriate for their own level of development: Bobby, a turtle puppet (Bobby asked therapist for it); Kathy, a pencil sharpener (child gave to therapist). Bobby's turtle from the therapist at his level of development represented a transitional object; Kathy's pencil sharpener to the therapist was related to the easing of her presenting problem of failure in school.

10   Both children showed growing feelings of love for therapist that were then reflected in relationships in external world, home and school.

11   Both showed increased capacity for learning.

The overall common element in the two therapies was the evidence of self-healing. Brian's and my joint description of the analytical process: "When the troubled child was protected in a free and safe container provided by the empathic therapist, the twin urges toward healing and growth set integrating functions of the psyche in motion."

Chapter 12

Child

Lucia Chambers

> The Soul that rises with us, our life's Star,
> Hath had elsewhere its setting,
> And cometh from afar:
> Not in entire forgetfulness,
> And not in utter nakedness,
> But trailing clouds of glory do we come
> From God, who is our home:
> Heaven lies about us in our infancy!
> William Wordsworth, from "Intimations of Immortality," 1807

Children have a mysterious power! When a toddler careens down the sidewalk, or a baby sitting on its mother's lap gurgles, or a child laughs in delight, all eyes are directed their way. Smiles touch many lips and the passerby pauses to be entranced. Producers of advertising know that the image of a baby, particularly the face and eyes, will catch the attention and soften the heart. When we look at a child, we can experience a glimmer of life as wondrous, filled with opportunities for fascinating new discoveries. Infinite possibilities, unlimited potential, and creativity – Wordsworth's "clouds of glory" – lie in the collective unconscious as the archetype of the child. The golden child, the magical child, the divine child are terms we use to refer to the great power that lies in the symbolic image of the child. Jung says that a child will arouse primitive longings in an adult for unfulfilled desires that have been lost in adaptation to civilization (Moore, 1992). A child reacts spontaneously and exuberantly, delights in expanding abilities to see more, touch more, taste more . . . be more. The child symbolizes the divine potential of creation, the ability to be more and more, pushing always toward our own totality, or the Self.

As well as the golden "clouds of glory," the child carries another aspect – that of abandonment. Jung describes the archetypal child as everything that is abandoned, exposed, vulnerable and yet divinely powerful (Moore, 1992). In myths and fairy tales, the child is lost in the forest, popped in an oven by a witch, eaten by a wolf, ostracized from the family or finds no room in the inn, even to be born. This special child is completely exposed to the vicissitudes of concrete reality. Many times, watching early scenes emerge in the sand, we see a baby or babies buried in the sand or lying lonely and helpless. There is a deep sense of loneliness, smallness and fear in these scenes, feelings that we try very hard to avoid or suppress. The aim of our system of education seems to be to hurry the child toward "growing out of it." We have graphs and charts that define "normal behavior," which is actually behavior that is quiet, conforming, and doesn't rock the boat, or it is the lesson plan of the day. Adults are critical of behavior that is childish or immature. We say, "Oh grow up!" when we cannot make sense of someone's attitude or behavior. In the sand room, adults are often embarrassed and confused when they are told they can play in the sand. "I don't know how; I feel stupid," one man said to me. And I knew that there was an abandoned, neglected, and perhaps even an abused child present in the room.

There is an increasing incidence and focus on abandoned, neglected and abused children. Today children are manifesting the neglect of the inner golden child and showing us rage, apathy and excesses of every kind. To reclaim that special inner child, with its joyous promise of aliveness, we need to be able to say, "I don't know" without shame. We must take in and acknowledge our own smallness and vulnerability. We must seek out the Zen "beginner's mind," because "Truly, I say to you, unless you turn and become like children, you will never enter the kingdom of heaven" (Mark 10:15).

Hillman comments in his foreword to Allan's book that there needs to be an escape from reasonable realism, backward and inward, to the inscapes of the child's soul – the restoring of the authenticity of the child's own visionary activity. These imaginary inscapes create a future reality, a reality that enlarges and deepens human consciousness (Allan, 1988). Sandplay invites one to enter those inscapes, into the vastness of imagination and fantasy, back into the vulnerability and wonder. After five years of weekly sandplay, a woman told me that she was not going to come to therapy any more. We had struggled together through her experience of ghastly sexual abuse starting at two years of age, numerous suicide attempts, rape, deep depression, and three bouts of cancer. Now she was facing a work-related disability. I wondered how she would keep going. We spoke on the phone periodically just so she could hear my voice and feel the continuity of our relationship. After about a year she reflected: "One day I was playing in the sand and I remembered *me*. The *me* that was there before all the awful stuff. And suddenly everything seemed so beautiful. And you were beautiful and the room was beautiful and the toys were beautiful, and I was beautiful. And I can still remember."

> Children should always show great forbearance toward grownup people.
>
> (St. Exupery, 1943, p. 17)

Part IV

Mother

Chapter 13

Mother trialogue

MARIA: My question is: What's the relationship between sandplay and mother? Why are we talking about mother?

KAY: If we go to Dora Kalff and Erich Neumann, one of the main challenges of development is the establishment of the mother–child unity within the individual psyche. A problem we may see in sandplay therapy, some place along the line, is that the mother–child unity hasn't been established. And to establish the Self, according to Neumann's and Kalff's theories, you have to have had an experience of mother–child unity.

MARIA: So you are saying that the mother–child relationship, with an experience of unity within that relationship, is essential in establishing the experience of the Self.

KAY: Yes. In sandplay, we will see some experience and expression of this mother–child relationship. When doing sandplay, a time will come when the sandplayer will put in a child and mother or a baby and a mother. Usually, when it first comes into the sandtray, it may be imaged as a mother and baby animal; or it is from a more distanced culture, like Asian or African; or it may be seen in the figures of gods and goddesses, such as the Virgin and Child. So this often comes in first, and then, as sandplayers keep working, they will begin to use figures from their own cultures. So, the mother is a very important part of sandplay.

LUCIA: The sand is important when we are talking about mother. The sand could represent the earth and the body . . .

MARIA: The body of the mother.

LUCIA: And mother. So, I think, the earth is the *prima materia*. Would that be prime material, Kay?

KAY: It's black material. *Prima* means the first, *prima materia* means the first material.

LUCIA: The *prima materia* as experienced through our hands touching the sand takes us back to the earth and to the mother.

MARIA: And the word "matter" comes from the Latin word "*mater*," which means mother.

KAY: I'd forgotten that. And touch is the first sensation that the baby has with the mother.

LUCIA: And don't you see people coming in and just touching the sand?

KAY: Or avoiding it.

LUCIA: Or avoiding it. Yes. That's right. So are sandplayers going towards the mother–child when they touch the sand, and then avoiding the mother when they do not want to touch the sand?

KAY: Yes, they're afraid of the mother–child experience. However, when you give sandplayers the good mother experience that they didn't have, or repeat what they did have, then this allows them to be able to touch the sand, and in touching the sand they are touching the earth. They can do this because they feel safe with you.

LUCIA: Early on, in some people's experience something about the safety has been broken.

KAY: Either broken or never established. And then, as sandplay therapists, we can establish or reestablish a feeling of safety by admiring and cherishing whatever the sandplayer does. And that's what a good mother does. And so that can give them an experience of good mothering.

LUCIA: Yup. So it's a going back, metaphorically, into the body of the mother. Isn't it? And then there's another birth, a birth of the Self, an experience of completion or wholeness.

KAY: Maybe not at first.

LUCIA: Yes, you have to go back down into the darkness and then, out again, into the light. If the unity with the mother was not adequately present, then the sandplayer may need the rebirth, because the ego has been damaged.

KAY: And the ego/Self axis hasn't been established.

LUCIA: That's right. So the relationship of the ego to the Self is damaged.

KAY: Or hasn't been established. I'm thinking about an article titled "Mommy and I are one," by Silverman [1985]. Two sets of psychiatric patients were presented with subliminal visual messages. The set for whom the message was "Mommy and I are one" showed a significantly greater decrease in pathology than the group who received a neutral message such as "It's a nice day." So it was the unconscious, without the conscious, that was experiencing the message of unity with the mother. I think that's pretty powerful.

LUCIA: And that is a tremendous requirement – or demand, then – of the sandplay therapist because, if we're not there on a subliminal level in a *totally* receptive way, then we repeat the wounding.

KAY: That's it. That happens in verbal therapy, too. It isn't just sandplay. That's the reason therapists have to do so much work on themselves. They've got to get to their own wounds.

LUCIA: Nevertheless, this seems easier for sandplay therapists – even though it's so hard. In verbal therapy – where we're always going back, "Well, tell me about your mother." And then there's this long dialogue for – it can be endless – session after session after session – about the pain, *and* the abandonment, the wounding. It just goes on forever in a verbal kind of way. It's hard to get out of it.

KAY: A therapist may get into it themselves verbally. And then they may get a negative transference/countertransference thing going.

MARIA: Sometimes in verbal therapy, there is the ability to get to the positive from the negative through empathic attunement.

KAY: Right. But then you're using a nonverbal tool; empathy is nonverbal.

MARIA: Right. You're in the realm of the nonverbal/preverbal. You're in the realm of responding emotionally and empathically to what is going on. Sometimes, when I am working, I can tell when someone's in the realm of the preverbal mother because the words that I'm saying don't matter. They are listening to the sound of my voice.

KAY: Right. Even though you are speaking, it's the voice that they hear, so you are in the nonverbal realm.

MARIA: Yes. They don't really remember what I'm saying but they're listening to the sound of my voice, and that is what is soothing to them. Here we are in the realm of the primal mother–child unity and we are responding from there.

LUCIA: We were talking before about the holding quality of sand and doing sand work, the holding of whatever the client brings. And it's that holding quality that's the maternal.

MARIA: Yes.

LUCIA: It's the holding, not the words. And when words are taken away from you and you can't use them any more, there may be a lot of fear and anxiety. People always try to go back to words but when the words are gone, then the drop happens into the nonverbal subliminal level. But maybe sometimes that isn't what people are willing to risk because at that time they can't go into the mother, or into the sand.

KAY: I always remember a woman who came to do sandplay. I didn't think that she was really relating to me but we went on. And then she put in a perfume bottle top. I had never seen it used any other way than as a crystal tree. So, when she put it in, I just thought it was like that. But later, when I asked her what it was, she said, "Oh, my mother used L'Heure Bleue perfume, too." So then I knew that she had been in the transference.

LUCIA: And – you didn't have to name that – and you didn't have to deal with it – directly.

KAY: But, of course, I didn't know this until we reviewed the sand scenes some time after the sandplay process had been completed.

LUCIA: She didn't tell you this at the time?

KAY: No. So, I just went on. What if I had asked her at the time, "What is that for?" I think that would have been bad. I do not think she could have let me know at the time that she was connected to me and relating to me that much.

LUCIA: No, she couldn't.

KAY: So it worked. And later, I could see how important it was for her to put in the perfume bottle top. It was an important experience of the transference in the tray.

MARIA: Yes. That's a lovely example of the co-transference.

LUCIA: It's beautiful. You didn't have to deal with it directly.

KAY: At the time – I didn't know what it was. But it didn't matter. See, this is the point. These things happen and we don't have to understand all the symbolization. And this is what a lot of sandplayers can't understand. They think they *should* understand what all the symbols mean. But the nonverbal works for them anyway – even though they don't know what the symbol means.

LUCIA: That's right.

MARIA: But you knew enough about the other symbols, and what was happening, and the feeling in the room. And you could hold her and what was happening to her –

KAY: I knew I liked her – very much. And I knew that she was in a process because I can tell when a person is in a process.

MARIA: That's what I mean. You understood that something very powerful was happening.

KAY: That's right, but I didn't understand that symbol. Or perhaps many others. But I – yeah, I knew that she was in a process. I knew that she was wounded. I knew that she was working hard and – and her psyche was going to do it. She came regularly. I knew it was work. It wasn't just the regularity. I knew from the trays that she was working, *it* was working.

MARIA: Right. And you could see that – even if you didn't sit there and think, "This means this and that means that," you could see this very profound unfolding of a process in what she was creating. You were in there with her.

KAY: I was in there with her but I want to emphasize the point that I didn't *have* to know all that. If she felt cherished by me, if she felt the cherishment, then she could go ahead. She knew that I was there, I was witnessing this. I didn't have to understand it.

LUCIA: No. I had an experience like that too. A woman with the most horrendous child abuse – just horrendous – came to do the sand. And there was a lot of stuff in the sand which I could be with without knowing about it. And she did sand without telling me a lot at first. I knew it was heavy because of – the darkness – of what I was seeing in the sand. But I could hold it. Then, when she went to the verbal part – after she felt comfortable and started telling me details – I had a lot of trouble holding it, a lot of trouble. It was too much!

KAY: Too painful.

LUCIA: Too awful! But I didn't have trouble in the sand. And she was very perceptive, and she said, "Now, I don't know if you want to hear this." And after the second session I said, "I don't know if I do, either. But the sand can hold it." And she said, "Yes, I know it can." So we went on. But there's something – the personal, the ego levels – are set aside in the sand – so that you can be Mother without the ego coming in and saying, "How could her mother do that to her?" And it made me realize how thankful I am for the sandtray.

KAY: You have had this experience in the sandplay. And so you know it – intimately and can work with her from this place of knowing.

LUCIA: Being a mother is not easy. It is *really* hard.

KAY: Challenging.

LUCIA: No, it's *hard*! And so giving that over to the sand is wonderful!

KAY: If a sandplayer can put a witch in the sand and cut its head off, they aren't saying to you directly that they want to cut your head off, but it is being held between you.

LUCIA: Or smashing some of those things with rocks.

KAY: Or pulling arms off my dear little witch that never got arms back again.

LUCIA: Yes, we are able to hold the most horrible experiences.

KAY: We can cherish the sandplayer more because they're not attacking us personally and yet we know that they are working it out in the sand.

LUCIA: That's right.

KAY: There are other examples of negative feeling expressed towards the mother in sand.

LUCIA: Well it is important to focus on what's in the sand closest to where the therapist is sitting.

MARIA: For example, a figure pointing a gun at the therapist is an obvious one; or a volcano placed close to the therapist.

LUCIA: Yes, that has to do with negative feeling towards the mother and it has to do with the therapist. But the therapist doesn't need to automatically sink into that role.

KAY: Absolutely. They have to cherish, and that is the function of the good-enough mother.

LUCIA: Yeah. Yeah.

KAY: My other story is of a young woman in her early twenties who came to me – she needed to be cherished. She had to be loved. And this went on for a long time. One day she came in and she said, "I don't have to have you mother me any more."

LUCIA: Oh!

KAY: "I want you to not just love me for myself. I want you to love me for what I can do. Like yesterday I took a test and I got a top score." So we changed. And I acquired the role of father. The first part of my therapy often is a mothering. But there comes to a time when you really have to change.

LUCIA: To more of the doing.

KAY: More of the doing. The father role is admiring the doing and the mother role is admiring you for yourself.

LUCIA: For being. I remember when I first started learning about psychology. It's the mother – everything comes from the mother and the mother is to blame for everything. And I hated that. But with sandplay, the mother – or the sand or the holding, the cherishing – *can* do everything. It can facilitate the change of the entire perceptual way of the sandplayer. It can, if you stay with the sand, the sand will hold it.

KAY: It may take a long, long, long time. And sometimes that is very discouraging. And so you think, "Well, I'll start talking. Maybe that would help." And it doesn't.

LUCIA: It doesn't help at all. It makes it go on longer even.

MARIA: I have a different experience. In the healing of my own mother wound, sandplay enabled me to have a nonverbal experience of holding and an experience of acceptance and being cherished for myself, which was really essential. But I also needed to have an analysis along with the sandplay to heal it.

LUCIA: A regular Jungian analysis, you mean? Is that what you mean?

MARIA: Yes, I needed the words. I have so much feeling about it. Something got touched in me in the sand that was what held the essence of the process of the analysis. But I needed a human being who could give verbal expression to the suffering. The sandplay was essential and wonderful but it wasn't enough – for me. I don't think I could have done it without the sandplay and the deep experience of holding on the nonverbal level. However, I needed to have the words of another expressing and understanding all that suffering, as well.

LUCIA: So, for you, sand – by itself – was not enough.

MARIA: It wasn't.

KAY: For me, analysis wasn't enough.

LUCIA: That's it. So it's –

MARIA: It's the combination.

LUCIA: There's some kind of a lovely combination and the therapist needs to be attuned to what is needed.

MARIA: For me it was a combination. I know that my analysis couldn't have gone where it went without the sandplay. But my analyst didn't do sandplay. So I did sandplay with somebody else.

LUCIA: It's the combination.

MARIA: Which is profound! And I don't know what it would have been like if my analyst had done sandplay.

KAY: No. One doesn't. One only knows one's own experience. Well, thank you. I appreciate your sharing that.

MARIA: I'm most struck by my deep feelings as you were talking. I was deeply touched by the discussion of the nonverbal mother–child connection.

I think that's why the sand can be so frightening to people. They touch it and it brings up so much feeling.

LUCIA: That is why I say to a sandplayer when they complete a tray, "Is there anything you need to say about this?," letting them know that words are fine. It's not that words are forbidden.

MARIA: Yeah.

LUCIA: In working with Dora, she put words into my work with her. She put words there – she pulled them out of somewhere else. She would say things that I was unconscious of and made me see what I had done in a totally different way.

KAY: Well, that's interesting. I suppose that was her skill in choosing whether to speak or not. With me, she didn't talk much. And for ten years I didn't know what had really happened in the trays because we didn't look at the trays I had created until then. And yet – yet it worked.

LUCIA: She didn't say anything about –

KAY: Not – not about the – the essence. Not about the most important part. And I didn't know about it for ten years, and yet it worked. You see, we have had completely different experiences and yet it has worked for each of us. So our experiences do color what we do in therapy. And a very important part of sandplay is the therapist. Their own experience and their ability to adjust to whatever is needed at the time is essential.

LUCIA: And isn't that the mother, as the mother has to be ready to play or to talk or to be quiet?

KAY: That is the good-enough mother.

LUCIA: That's right. She – and she doesn't get to decide. The baby decides.

MARIA: The good-enough mother has to be attuned and responsive.

KAY: And I would say that the sandplayer decides pretty much, too.

LUCIA: You have to be really tuned in to what the sandplayer is wanting or needing. That's a good point, Maria, about not saying you can't talk or everything has to be nonverbal. It is some kind of a beautiful ebb and flow that looks different for everyone . . . for every single person it looks different.

MARIA: But sandplay touches us at that profound level of the nonverbal – of the first relationship before there were words. Then as therapists we're touched by that and we respond.

LUCIA: That's right.

KAY: And I also give credit to the psyche in determining what it needs. It will push the therapist aside if that's what's needed. I'm always amazed at how the psyche will reach out for what it needs.

LUCIA: Mm-hmm. I've always found that words get everything all scrambled in my head. So, for years of Jungian analysis, it was just a mess in there – a big scrambled mess. I understood. But it didn't heal me. And the sand just did it because it got down below my mind. And then the wonderful thing – and maybe this is what you're talking about – is that, after the sand did whatever it did, then the verbal analysis *really* caught hold. So there must have been some – someplace I went to where I found what I needed without knowing what I needed and then I could bring it up and use it again, verbally. But it was also the combination.

KAY: Coming back to the mother, we might talk about how mother is seen in various ways in the tray.

LUCIA: She comes into the process in a lot of different ways.

KAY: And even after you've seen hundreds and hundreds of trays, you still see another new way she may come in. But after seeing hundreds of trays, you are more aware that something in the tray is a mother thing and you can appreciate it.

LUCIA: The mother even comes in through the hands of the client sometimes. You can tell if they're very gentle and soft and – and then it's comforting when you see that softness come in around the figures – and the delicateness of it. It's – it's the – the mother's spirit, I think, being very careful and –

KAY: Often we see breasts in the sand.

MARIA: Or a belly mound in the sand.

KAY: One woman I saw – when we were going to be separated because of our vacations – made two breasts. And I knew and she knew what this meant. Even though she had not wanted to be too dependent on me. She then made a third one and then a fourth one and put nipples on all four. These individual experiences are always amazing to me.

MARIA: The formations in the sand are important connections to the mother and the mother–child co-transference: the breasts, the mounds – for the belly, pregnant bellies or even a whole torso of the mother, in the sand.

LUCIA: It is body.

MARIA: Also cave-like spaces that are closed and contained, these are powerful mother symbols, or images.

LUCIA: The sand itself is an important part of the sandtray.

KAY: And the water, when the sandplayer gets to using water.

LUCIA: Trays with rice or beans don't have the same pull down. Don't you think? It has to be earth.

KAY: Or people that think they can do it without any tray, just on a table. Then there's no container and no sand or water.

MARIA: Another phenomenon I have noticed is when sandplayers put something in the tray that is related to your mother or theirs, for example the perfume bottle top. I remember a nine-year-old girl who lost her mother when she was five. In the very first tray, she picked up some black beads that *my* mother had given *me* and she put them into the tray. And so we were right in the mother work.

KAY: That's that mystical stuff. That must have touched you.

MARIA: I was immediately attuned to her at that level, right from the get-go. This little girl was focused on achievement and would only talk about her achievements in school. She would just chatter away and didn't want to talk about her mother dying, didn't want to talk about her feelings. It was too scary. But when she went to the sandtray, she worked. She worked and worked – and did not speak. She would do it for the whole session. And that's where she expressed herself and experienced her grief and loss and mourned the death of her mother. Then we'd play cards and have chatty little conversations. But the work, the mother work, was in that tray.

KAY: You could separate them.

LUCIA: Isn't that lovely?

MARIA: And this was a case where there was never any discussion about her mother dying. But she could mourn her mother through the sandplay.

KAY: And she felt safe.

LUCIA: And that is the mother work and I told you mother is work.

Chapter 14

Mother

Maria Ellen Chiaia

When focusing on the personal and archetypal realms of the mother there is much for sandplay to learn and integrate from infant observation and developmental, analytic theory (Jacoby, 1999; Fordham, 1970). Sandplay touches, at a profound level of the nonverbal, our first relationship with mother, before there were words. As sandplay therapists this realm is touched through feelings and emotions that are stirred in the sandplayer and us when a person is creating a sandtray. We respond to these feelings empathically; there is an emotional attunement that occurs nonverbally. From this attunement to this maternal realm of the preverbal, images and thoughts arise from these earliest relationships. Sandplay provides a space for the expression and then experience of these realms between therapist and sandplayer. These places are shared and metabolized by the therapist.

Since the development of the ego–Self axis begins preverbally in a mother–infant environment of being, there is real power and beauty in the nonverbal experience of an imaginal process within a relationship between therapist and client. Transformation occurs in silence at the level of being where the interpersonal unconscious meets at the level of the Self in a field. Infant observation and research show that the relationship between the mother and infant is key in the transformational process of growth of ego and its relationship to the Self. The maternal caregiver provides a continuity of being in her holding and presence. There is an aesthetic of being that is created by the mother in how she handles and relates to her infant. The sandplay therapist meets the sandplayer in this place of being and the aesthetic creation of the sandplayer mirrors this transformational experience. The process of transformation is set in motion and processes that alter the ego and Self are experienced.

The ability of the sandplayer to approach the sand and to engage the sand is all part of this realm. Other aspects of this maternal realm include how the sandplayer touches the sand, what is created in the sand, and what forms and shapes appear in the sand. All of these experiences evoke feelings in the therapist and sandplayer. According to Balint (1999), and as stated in Chapter 6, feeling is correlated with touching and associated with our most primary object relations, which are created and maintained through interaction between two people by nonverbal means. In this realm of the primal mother–child unity, the therapist is responding emotionally and empathically to what is going on and so is the client. Even if there are words, it is the sound of the therapist's voice and the quality of emotion being expressed that become important.

The following case of a nine-year-old girl, Sandy, who lost her mother illustrates the material above. Developmental issues emerged and then arrested development resumed as Sandy worked with issues of the loss of her mother. Her experience during sandplay was one of transformation and inspiration as she faced death, mourned, found a connection to the lost mother and then found herself in life, reconnected to her inner world.

My understanding of the co-transference was informed through silence and the unspoken communications that passed between us. Sandy spoke very little, sometimes not even saying hello or goodbye. She would go directly over to the tray where she worked with great seriousness and focus for the whole hour. Strong feelings would come and go in me but Sandy expressed very little feeling during the two years that I saw her. When she did speak it was brief and superficial and her affect seemed stilted and dead. However, when she was doing a sandtray, her feelings were alive and engaged.

I came to understand that beneath a calm surface, Sandy's currents ran powerful and deep. Sandy needed me to be present, and allow plenty of space and silence so that she could integrate the powerful emotions she experienced in doing the sandplay. I saw Sandy as a private child unable to discuss her thoughts and feelings with another. However, in the large spaces of silence, Sandy was able to experience what was buried and that allowed her to find life again.

At the time of Sandy's first session it had been barely three years since her mother's death. One year previously, Sandy had lost the house she grew up in with her mother and all that they owned was lost: pictures, jewelry, toys and familiar objects.

In her initial tray (Figure 14.1), the nature of the problem and the issues to be worked appeared. Sandy began by smoothing the sand and then she dug three holes and sprayed water in these holes. She buried rocks or jewels in the sand and sprinkled water to indicate where these things were buried. Water, the source of life, was used now and in subsequent trays to mark and protect what had been hidden or lost.

She put in four pyramids, Egyptian tombs used to bury the pharaohs and much of what they would need in the next world. Perhaps Sandy felt as if she had been buried along with her dead mother and felt lifeless and lost. She connected a string of black beads from one of the pyramids to the water holes. She seemed to be protecting this main source of water, her source of life, by encircling and connecting it to the crystal pyramid. Since this was the only crystal pyramid in the tray it may have had some special significance.

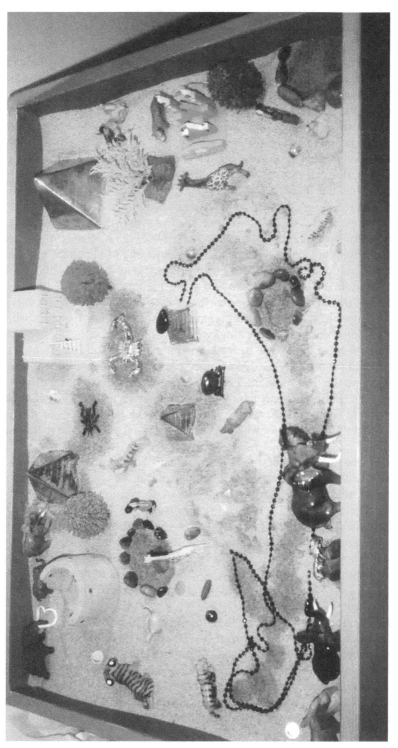

Figure 14.1 A tray by Sandy

Maybe it showed where her mother was buried. The presence of the mother in the transference between us is suggested by Sandy's use of the string of black beads that belonged to my own mother.

In the corner of the tray nearest to where I sit, there is a wet hole with jewels buried in it. Also there is a vessel and a woman with a vessel. Given this configuration as well as the way Sandy responded to my questions with silence, I imagine that at the time she unconsciously wanted me to hold a space for her: a silent container that would allow Sandy to be alone in my presence so that she could eventually find a relationship to the mother that had been lost and that she needed to find.

There are five tigers in this tray. Tigers need a home range of between eight and forty square miles and maintain exclusive rights to this home range. To survive they need to kill a large animal weighing between one hundred and four hundred pounds every five to eight days. When these ecological requirements are not met the overcrowded tigers come in contact with people and livestock and hunt them (Macdonald, 1987).

In this sandtray there is an overcrowding of tigers. Sandy may have felt threatened by these large predatory forces within her and/or she may have felt hungry and unsatisfied due to the loss of her mother. This unsatisfied hunger may have resulted in uncontained aggression and rage within her with no internal "good" mom to help contain these "bad" forces. The giraffes, the young girl, the woman and baby, the woman, and the elephants are all vulnerable. They are all competing for the limited supplies of food and water. This is not a "benign environment" (Winnicott, 1965).

The solution may be found in the kiva (Figure 14.1, upper left), an Indian ceremonial structure built into the earth, where tribal initiations of life and death are enacted. As we will see in the following trays, Sandy had the developmental task of losing and finding the mother so that some sense of object constancy could be attained. She needed to go into the earth over and over again as she buried and unburied her dead mother and the archetypal mother. She needed to experience the split-off feelings and thereby gain mastery and control of what had occurred in her nine years of life. The kiva as well as the church (Figure 14.1, right middle) may be symbolic of the meaning and working through of life and death issues.

Throughout the sandtray series that Sandy created, she buried the figures she used in her trays and then used an object to dig up the items she buried in the sand. Sometimes she just left them buried. It is important to note that this kind of play, prevalent in games of peek-a-boo with very young children, begins the developmental task of separation from the mother. According to Winnicott (1965), only when children have achieved some sense of constancy and continuity in the world around them can they tolerate some separation from those they love and depend on. Therefore children become able to tolerate separation from parts of themselves to which they have become disconnected. After losing and finding over and over, object constancy is eventually attained. Sandy's early losses disrupted this development. By feeling and touching the sand, Sandy was experiencing the feeling and touching that was connected to her earliest relating with the mother of her infancy.

In many of her trays, after she buried and dug up and buried, Sandy left the sandtray in a devastated and destroyed state. Perhaps she was experiencing the feelings that she had felt when her mother had left her by dying. As she practiced and played at losing and finding, she needed to destroy and to find the split-off parts she had lost. Upon her return each week to the playroom and the sandtray, she found the tray had survived her destruction. At that point she purposely returned to losing and finding.

In tray two (Figure 14.2), there is a devastated look and feel to the tray. There is the feather that she used as the object to dig and find the buried figures. There is a reappearance of pyramids, three this time. She placed two totems, perhaps the continued representation of the native culture as seen in tray one. The ceremonial nature of her task was to find a deeper connection to family and Self, as totem poles are emblems of family or clans signifying ancestral relationships. The carved images represent the family's or tribe's kinship or mystical relationship with the animals or symbols depicted.

In tray four Sandy buried a treasure chest in a cave. She then closed up the cave by building a mountain on top of it. In the mountain, Sandy buried and dug up many figures: warriors, skeletons, coffins, pennies, a crystal ball, a broom, a magician, and a toucan. She uncovered everything with a broom, which she found, and then reburied everything, flattening the scene and leaving it.

During the making of this tray, she worked with furious determination. As she worked, I was filled with grief. I imagine that I was feeling all of what she felt but dared not utter. She rang a bell once during the process, alerting me to the ritualistic aspect of her play, preparing both of us for the transformation, which would occur in the following tray.

When this tray was completed, she asked for some plasticine clay and created a bright, colorful bird. The bird is a hopeful symbol and it has food and water, emotional and psychological nourishment (A. Mazzarella, personal communication, 1993). Sandy needed hope and nourishment. Like the bell, this bird was preparing both of us for the following tray. Birds are viewed as symbols of death and rebirth and are connected with goddesses of death and transformation (Neumann, 1963; Johnson, 1988). From the earliest times when associated to the Great Mother, birds have appeared as symbols of death and rebirth.

After working through the devastating loss and surviving it, working with the issues of mother–child unity, we come to a Self tray (Figure 14.3). The client's Self tray revealed the appearance of the central organizing principle inherent in the psyche. This is not to be confused with a healthy ego that can

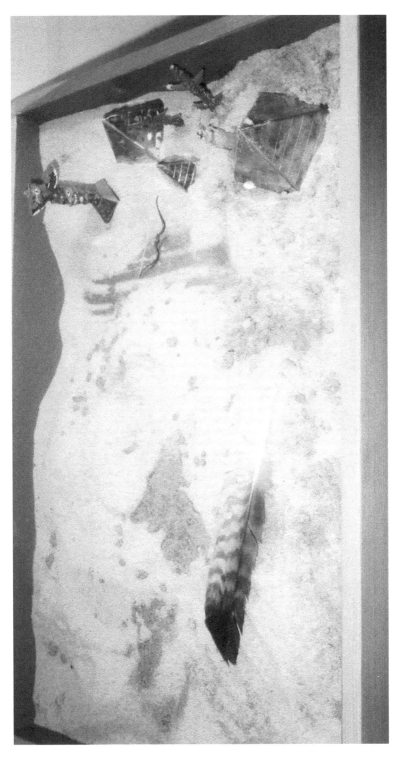

Figure 14.2 A tray by Sandy

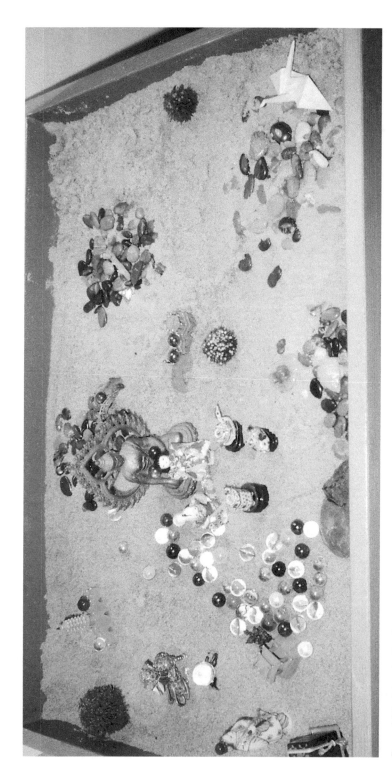

Figure 14.3 A tray by Sandy

organize and master the world in a conscious way. First note how naturally clear and organized this tray is, as compared to the other trays I have discussed. The organization of the tray itself suggests the Self at work in connection to Sandy's intact ego. Here we see the ego–Self connection for the first time.

In the center of this tray there is the appearance of a central historical manifestation of the Self, the Buddha. Buddha is the supreme manifestation of compassion and unity in the world of suffering, and he is accompanied by two divine children, also representatives of the birth of the Self. They protect and preside over all the jewels and stones that she had been burying and digging up for three weeks. The jewels have been found and are shown.

There are also temples, and a few trees, which are either flowering or full of fruit. There are also three beautiful containers and a temple guardian. Here we see an origami (folded paper) crane, another bird. Johnson states that cranes, birds of rebirth, are symbols of life. Sandy had certainly returned from the death and destruction she had visited over the previous years. She played the music box. She seemed peaceful and happy after this tray.

Having found inner wholeness, for a moment, in the following sessions she returned again to the burying and digging up; but this time there were new figures to which she needed to attend. Sandy made five trays like this. With time they became more and more sparse as she picked up the work of burying and digging.

In this series, however, she created some solid land formations, mountains and volcanoes and an interesting land formation. In a later tray, she put a *sipapu*, which is a place of emergence. Native American creation myths tell of the place deep in the earth where the ancestors lived, and from where they emerged whole through the *sipapu*, thus initiating life on earth.

After a summer break, Sandy returned and was sad and quiet. She started by mixing water and sand and then buried Hawaiian musicians, dancers and marbles, layering them in the sand. She made a mound over the layered figures and then made a cross on top. She seemed to be creating a large grave. She placed a mother and a daughter on the mound.

This is the first time that there was the appearance of two humans that are close to her identity as they are a white mother and daughter. They were having a picnic. She played the music box, which plays the "Teddy Bears' Picnic." She buried and dug with the feather and then put in the figures and the feather. Amid all this devastation and work, on top of the buried figures and jewels, there was a sharing of food, a symbol of nurturance and care.

Sandy seemed to be reconnecting to these qualities and feelings within her which had disappeared with her mother. I felt a warm connection to Sandy. I imagined she was experiencing with me a deep silent communion as she worked with devastation and loss.

In the spiral she drew in the sand and another spiral she created with the jewels, there again was a pattern of wholeness and the inner ordering principle of the Self. We also see the movement of the spiral (Chambers, 1990), which could be an expression and honoring of her journey into the land of the dead – to her mother's residence.

After the second manifestation of the Self, in the form of a spiral, lined with marble jewels, Sandy returned to normal life and the ordinariness of daily living. In one of her final trays a house was set up for Christmas and then in the next tray a house was set up for a dinner party. In both scenes there was food on the table. Sandy had found the food and sustenance she had been needing and this sustaining nourishment was finally safe and contained in ordinary life.

In the next to last tray, Sandy returned to the Native American Indian motif from the first tray. This time there were no tigers. There were lots of sources of food. The kiva is buried deeper. There is a toy oven and three more ovens that she created with the sand. The ovens, places for cooking, are perhaps symbolic of her ability to obtain warmth and nurturance by transforming raw substances, her raw feelings of hunger and rage, into something edible and nurturing. Two kachinas, different manifestations of spiritual forces, the forces of life and death, are present in this tray. Certainly Sandy had worked with these forces throughout the making of her sandplay pictures.

In the final tray (Figure 14.4), she put the stone jewels in her everyday world. They were among houses and cars, and again a picnic is set. The black beads from the first tray are surrounding a ferryboat. Perhaps this was Charon's ferry that crosses the river Styx into the world of the dead, and maybe it had retrieved Sandy from the land of the dead. She had needed to go there to find the lost parts of herself, as well as the jewel of the Self that had disappeared with her mother.

Through the nonverbal empathic attunement of the co-transference, Sandy experienced the primary object relations connected to touching and feeling as she touched objects and sand belonging to me as well as connecting to the mother earth through the sand and water. By returning to the experience of mother–child unity, she found a deep connection to ego, to Self and other, and having found them obtained the constancy and continuity that was missing. Having found them, she was able to be herself, separate and unique. We see this sense of identity in her footprint, which she imprinted in the sand. She created it by pressing her sneaker in the sand (Figure 14.4). Sandy had arrived.

This case illustrates how play, developmental themes and transformation are dynamically interrelated with the experience of mother–child unity and the archetypal Self. By losing and finding over and over again in the sand, Sandy found object constancy and therefore a more secure sense of herself. Throughout this work her connections to the Mother and to the archetypal Self were also found.

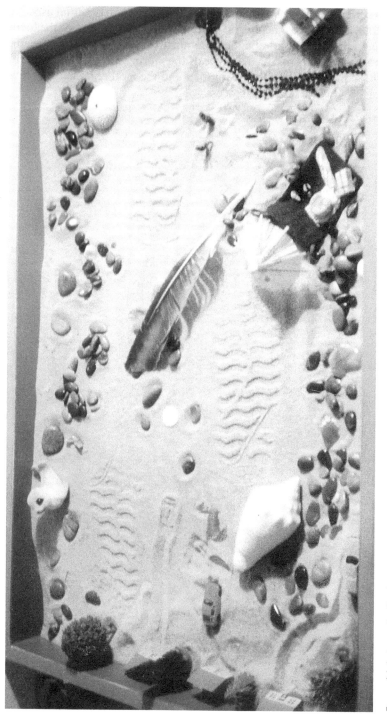

Figure 14.4 A tray by Sandy

This experience of mother–child unity and the Self is an essential aspect of any sandplay experience. Facing and experiencing some aspects of the loving and hating, comforting and abandoning, nurturing and depriving, creating and destroying, aspects of the archetype of the mother are important for any individuation process. The personal mother and the mother archetype are an essential aspect of any sandplay process.

Chapter 15

Mother

Kay Bradway

The mother plays many roles in all therapies of the psyche. I have selected just three of these roles to focus on here: mother–child unity, or the initial relationship between mother and infant; mothering, or a client's struggle with negative feelings toward her own child; mother projection, or the transferring of both positive and negative images toward one's mother onto one's therapist.

Mother–child unity

One of the first symbol meanings I recall hearing from Dora Kalff was "mother–child unity." Other Jungian analysts have referred to the relationship between mother and child, or "mother–child relationship," but Kalff was the first one to recognize the earliest bonding between mother and baby as a "unity." I am reminded of the research of Lloyd Silverman in which the subliminal message of "Mommy and I are one" had a significant influence on the subsequent attitude and behavior of the subjects (Silverman, 1985). These findings reflect the power of that initial relationship, unity, with the mother.

Dora Kalff's referring to "mother–child unity" in her classes alerted us to look for its appearance in the sandplay pictures – at first in her cases, and then in those presented by others in her classes. It was always a recognition that the sandplay process was under way when an image placed in the sand could be identified as an image of mother–child unity.

Kalff describes the term "mother–child unity" as a psychological concept in the opening paragraphs of her book on sandplay. She writes: "When all of the requirements of a newborn infant, such as appeasement of hunger, shelter from cold, etc., are met by the bodily mother, the child experiences an unconditional security and a sense of safety through motherly love. We call this first phase the *mother–child unity*" (2003, p. 1, emphasis in original).

Kalff saw the Self as initially being contained within the mother and later separating from her. She writes: "After one year, the Self of the child – the center of his psychic totality – separates itself from the Self of the mother . . . A relationship of trust grows out of this experience" (2003, pp. 1–2).

Mother–child unity may be seen in many different images. I have found that it is often first shown in images representing other cultures than one's own, or in animal figures, or in mythological figures. These can come before sandplayers are able to use a mother–child combination that is closer to their own outer experience.

In understanding the meaning of mother figures in the tray, one has to be alert to both the commonly associated meaning and the biological reality. An example is the alligator, which in my experience is commonly associated with the image of a devouring mother, and therefore a negative mother. The biological reality is that alligators are very good mothers; they actually help their babies in hatching from the eggs and in making their way to the river. There are pictures of alligator mothers transporting their babies in their mouths to the river. I wonder if the false association of alligator with devouring mother might have come from babies in mothers' mouths being interpreted as babies being devoured by their mothers.

Mothering

Although sandplay is usually used by sandplayers to work on their relation-ships with their own mothers, sometimes a woman will use sandplay to work on herself as a mother, on mothering. Rhoda provides an example.

When Rhoda started her sandplay process, she was having problems with her baby daughter. Her initial scene included an athlete beside a crying baby with a black mask below them. She said the athlete represented the strength she needed to wrestle with the baby and that the black mask represented her rage. In the review she explained, "At that time I was just discovering my rage."

As her first placement in the next tray, Rhoda put an Eskimo mother with her baby. She described the placement as giving her a feeling of collective mothering. She observed, "It gives me a feeling of reuniting with all that. It was both a personal mother, I, and my child, but also the universal mother and child." She added objects that represented her relation with her own mother, reflecting the experience of a mother-line, which is so important to mothers, especially with their first babies. As if to reinforce the feeling of mothering, Rhoda added a kangaroo with its baby, and an Indian squaw with a baby.

The next trays showed further development of Rhoda's relationship with her baby daughter to a rewarding and loving closeness. In her final tray she placed a large and a small starfish near to each other but clearly separated from one another. She indicated that they represented herself and her baby daughter. After going from rage toward her child to a feeling of love, she was now able to experience closeness to, but separation from, her baby. This process is consistent with Kalff's descriptions of changes in the mother–child relationship – here from the point of view of a mother (Bradway and McCoard, 1997, p. 170).

Mother projection

Projecting of negative feelings toward one's own mother onto one's therapist is probably a necessary stage in depth therapy. In fact it may provide for a recognition of "depth therapy" in that it takes one back and down to the very depth of one's psyche. A therapist's experience of being loved by a client may pose problems. Experiences of being hated by a client may cause problems and often cause genuine pain. But it is an understandable part of the therapeutic relationship. After all, therapists both give and withhold. They hold power just as mothers do. They provide protection, but on their terms. They limit the time; they ask for payment; they abandon you when they take vacations. A client's anger may be a necessary part of the relationship. Sandplay offers a way in which the rage can be expressed and experienced by both client and therapist without threat to the therapist. Emmy's sandplay process provides an example.

After Emmy portrayed herself and her therapist, me, in the first tray as if headed on a path toward a common goal, things went smoothly in the relationship until there was a misunderstanding about an appointment time. Such misunderstandings can cause feelings of guilt and resentment in both client and therapist. Whose fault was it? Then I was late for the next appointment, an unconscious acting out on my part. It came out later that Emmy had been enraged by multiple experiences of others being late. So this did it! She made me wait before she put anything into the sandtray. Then for the first time she put in aggressive images: a crusader brandishing a sword, fire, a dragon. I was not hurt, but she could experience her rage and communicate it to me through the sandplay, rather than risking communicating it in words, which at that time she was not ready to do. In fact she never did use words to express anger towards me. She did not have to use words. She could experience it in the sandplay process. And it was after she made the tray with fire and killing that she made a scene in which the figure she identified as herself was seated by an open treasure box. Emmy carefully removed a crystal from the box and placed it by the woman figure.

Michael Fordham once told me that he did not like to use sandplay because he wanted the patient to see the witch (the bad mother) in him, not in an image in the tray. But sandplay does not preclude seeing the witch in the therapist. Emmy saw the witch in me as well as in the tray, but she could work most of it out in the trays without having to attack me in person. And then in the protection of the therapeutic relationship she could attain the treasure (Bradway and McCoard, 1997, pp. 199–200).

Chapter 16

Mother

Lucia Chambers

> The mother stands for the collective unconscious, the source of the water of life.
>
> (Jung, 1968a, par. 92)

"In the beginning" in the consciousness of the earliest human, there was a profound awareness of the cyclic nature of life and all its many forms. Light followed dark, birth followed death, wet followed dry, cold followed hot, each element in relation to and dependent upon the existence of the other. There was a majestic, mystical "oneness" of all life.

This oneness became associated with the female body in that She carries death in her monthly cycle of bleeding, and also carries life in the great Round of her belly and sustains that life with nourishment from her own body. Neumann says:

> The Feminine appears as great because that which is contained, sheltered, nourished, is dependent on it and utterly at its mercy. Nowhere perhaps is it so evident that a human being must be experienced as "great" as in the case of the mother. A glance at the infant or child confirms her position is Great Mother ... We arrive at a universal symbolic formula for the early period of mankind: Woman = body = vessel = world.
>
> (1963, p. 43)

The absolute power for the existence of the world rested in the feminine; she became She, became sacred, became God/Goddess. Her powerful symbols are still found in myths, art, religion and music. She is suggested by containers of any kind. Figuratively she can be a country, the church, the city, the university, the spiral and the circle. Literally she is enclosures: the cave, a mound, houses and ships, pots, an oven, a ring, an egg, the sea. She is that which is fertile, such as animals (the cow and pig) and vegetation (the garden, corn and wheat). She is multiplicity.

As millennia went by, the evolution of human consciousness demanded more differentiation and discernment of these mysteries. Logos was rising. Early thinkers, including the alchemists, carried forward the idea of a single, original source. They postulated that before there was anything, before there was form, there was only undifferentiated matter or chaos.

This undifferentiated, single mass was called first matter or the *prima materia*. The Great Mother lost her form and became formless or chaotic, now available for exploration and therefore change. Her dominance as the regressive pull back to the womb and the instinctual level of existence had to be broken. Separation had to be struggled for if new life forms were to evolve. Jung saw this as the sacrifice of the animal nature in us, which fights against the urge toward individuation (1968b) but it is absolutely necessary in this stage of human consciousness. The theme of separation from the mother has been, and continues to be, a major issue for people of all cultures and races and brings much pain and struggle. It is perhaps the main topic of most psychoanalyses.

Individuation and development require the son to leave his mother, but he loves her and unconsciously longs for her all his life. Sometimes he requires similar qualities in the woman he marries, to her absolute frustration. The incestual, regressive pull urges a return to the mother and can trigger a desperate need to escape Her, which can bring about terrible wounding of both mother and son. The daughter too must leave the mother. Since the connection is like-to-like, the mother–daughter separation can be a powerful struggle. To foster this ripping apart, a violent masculine energy can emerge between mother and daughter, violating their unity. As in the myth of Demeter and Persephone there can be rape, victimization, death and sacrifice. When the daughter feels violated and abused by the realities of life, she might long for the unconscious safety and innocence of the virgin and declare she is "going home to Mother."

The separation from the mother is a developmental stage of every living creature. The human species, though, has a very tough time of it. We are the only species whose consciousness has a spiritual dimension, a connection with a nonmaterial reality. In order to develop this awareness and bring it into consciousness, we need the ego. The ego's function is to differentiate out the uniqueness of each individual's objective reality, to develop a separate personality out of the dark, uroboric oneness. Encoded in the psyche is an urge toward the light, toward order, toward Logos. It has pushed us, as a planet, as a civilization and as individuals into the state of patriarchal consciousness.

Patriarchal consciousness (not men and women) is explained by Neumann as consciousness coming from "the standpoint that the spirit is eternal *a priori*; that the spirit was in the beginning" (1963, p. 58). Now, with this leap, matter or Mater is pushed into secondary status. As patriarchal consciousness develops, it takes a position firmly in opposition to the instinctual wisdom held by the unbroken connection of the feminine bound to the earth and its cyclic destiny. Neumann expresses this shift:

> The victory of the male lies in the spiritual principle, which devaluates [sic] the moon and the feminine elements to which it belongs . . . and the soul which stands in opposition to the "pure spirit" . . . of the Apollonian–Platonic and Jewish–Christian form that . . . has led to the hypertrophy of consciousness at the expense of the whole man.
>
> (1963, p. 57)

This fundamental shift at the center of consciousness split the archetypal mother apart. That which was matter was relegated to the shadow. Matter, the human body and its functions, came to be seen as ugly, disgusting, dirty, and therefore in constant need of cleaning up or shunning. Chaos was too dark and vast to trust that any form would naturally be created out of it. So darkness and mutability went into the shadow. But paradoxically, that which was unchangeable, implacable and impersonal, resisting control and manipulation, also went into the shadow. Feeling, intuition and instinctual responses upset the order, and triggered undesirable experiences of helplessness and fear. So those too went into the shadow. Now, we have a huge shadowy mother who permeates every aspect of our lives. We have the Bad Mother.

The Bad Mother has been available and convenient to us to explain any of our pathological symptoms, large or small. She has appeared for thousands of years in demonic form in myths and legends. Lilith, from Kabbalistic tradition, creeps about at night in raw sexuality, then birthing 100 children every day and eating them as well as any human child she can snatch. Durga or black Kali, the Hindu Great Mother, forever lost in blood lust, tears the flesh from the bodies and wears the skulls as a necklace. Medea killed her sons in order to deprive her hated husband of his progeny. Hecate kills as she entangles one in her spells and incantations . . . or Astarte, or Circe, or Coatlicue. These are all personifications of the aspects of the Great Mother which have been split off and become demons and witches. The personal mother has been ruptured with this split by her mother and passes it on to her child, who passes it on, generation to generation. Every human child is wounded when it meets the "humanness" of its mother, that is the experience of a mother who does not act strictly in accordance with the child's needs. This is experienced as deprivation and rejection, needed in the natural order of development, but in our present context considered "bad." This failure can be relatively small, leaving behind neurosis or a mother complex, or it can be major, damaging the development of the ego and possibly leading to psychosis.

Every woman/mother carries Gaia within her psyche, but only the creative, supportive, nurturing aspects are welcomed into expression. All others are "bad" and the culture demands that they should be repressed. All shadowy reflections must be denied and compensated for. Mothers who talk with me wonder what they have done wrong. Maybe they didn't play enough, maybe they disciplined too hard, maybe they should have . . . done something differently. Even the "good-enough mother" implies failure of some kind. So, the child is angry with the mother and projects upon her all manner of the world's troubles. The mother is angry with herself and can treat the child as the instrument of her imprisonment and denial. The child is ashamed and abandons the child within. The mother is ashamed and abandons the fullness of her own psyche. She is not the "good" mother.

The perfection of the good mother, as defined by Logos, has created the archetype of Mary, Mother of God. She is the Mother of Light. In other words, she gives birth to the spirit. She does this only in relationship with God, who is self-conceiving, leaving her still virgin. She has no need of the body and all its messiness and decay. She is not bothered by hormones or moods. She is spirit without matter, light without dark. She has been so successfully split off from daily life that she cannot be manifested by mothers, by fathers or by the child.

Perhaps the primal wound that mars the development of the psyche is not only that the individual has been wounded by the personal bad mother, but that the experience of the totality of the Great Mother has not been incorporated into the universal consciousness. We are all thus wounded by her continued dissection and remain split within.

Redemption of the Feminine, that is, the totality of the Great Mother, within both men and women, is a concept that is becoming increasingly compelling. Hillman summarizes Jung in pointing out that "matter and spirit can no longer be such polar extremes, because the dogma [that is the dogma of the Assumption] heralds their union" (1972, p. 216). The perspective of the collective psyche will thus be transformed as well as the perception and experience of the personal feminine.

Dora Kalff said, "Reactivation of the feminine may be the way to activate the spirit. Centuries of neglect of feminine reality has led to the desiccation of spirit; rigidity and dogma. Our deepest religious impulses have been thwarted" (Weinrib, 1983, p. 41).

Kalff also felt that digging and working with the sand in the process of sandplay was an active way of encountering and working with the energies of the feminine, of reconnecting with the primal ground of our existence, with Gaia. We have all seen, many times, the symbolic images of the Dark Mother: skulls, graves, skeletons, witches, monsters, coffins, and blood. We have volcanoes and ice, snakes and crocodiles, and all manner of things black. We tend to see this darkness as the failure of the personal mother but it could also be the conscious identity of the split-off "Bad Mother" made available for potential union with her light counterpart. Jung says, "One does not become conscious by imagining figures of light but by making the darkness conscious" (1968c, par. 335). In these scenes filled with the darkness, if you look very carefully, you might see a hint of the coming of light. A bird, a little green thing, a bit of water, a tiny animal, a pearl, something gold. Psychic totality in the form of the Great Mother is there.

A new creative psychology is emerging. Hillman declares, "The heroic age in psychology is past . . . The end of analysis coincides with the acceptance of femininity" (1972, p. 292). We are involved in "the compulsive search for psychic relatedness . . . We cannot go it alone . . . we must have a 'knowing together' "(p. 292).

And so we "are with" and hold the totality of the client as the sand holds the totality of us both.

> When after many years
> The daughter of her daughter
> Was searching for her homeland
> The rotten table
> Had prepared the soil for the fig tree seedling.
>
> In the centre of the former house
> She found a tree
> Rooted in the room
> Of her mother's mother.
> > Linde von Keyserlingk, 1992, p. 9

Part V

Self

Chapter 17

Self trialogue

MARIA: The Self cannot be represented.

KAY: You mean it cannot be represented by words. But can't it be represented by images?

MARIA: The archetype of the Self is unrepresentable. But it can be seen in or experienced in images.

KAY: Right. That's a good word, "experienced."

MARIA: It can be experienced but it isn't expressed in words.

KAY: No. There isn't a word for it. That's the reason we have so much trouble with it. We talk about Self trays and Self-constellation and Self-manifestation.

MARIA: And images of the Self as they appear in dreams and in the sand.

KAY: I was encouraged when I realized there was a difference between psyche and Self because I had used them both interchangeably. And I see why I did now – after talking with both of you. It's because the Self – it's like a god. It's something that is universal and we can't know it. We can talk about psyche as the whole, the totality, of an individual – the conscious and the unconscious.

MARIA: And that's different from the Self? And how would you say it was different if the psyche includes everything?

KAY: The psyche is the conscious and the unconscious, and it provides for the development of wholeness, which is supposedly the Self. But I think the Self must be there always.

MARIA: Well, I think the Self is what is guiding the process, at the deepest level of the psyche.

KAY: Well, okay. It depends on theory. If the Self doesn't come in until three years of age, such as Neumann and Dora Kalff say, then it cannot be that the psyche and the Self are the same.

LUCIA: No.

MARIA: I was saying that the Self is involved in the self-healing as part of the sandplay process.

KAY: After it comes in, it is. But, in the very beginning, it's the psyche that goes for healing, I think. Perhaps the psyche is like the acorn.

LUCIA: Are we talking about psyche as being an individual thing and the component of that particular individual's psyche? The Self is present all the time in all things and all psyches.

KAY: And the Self is more universal.

MARIA: Are you saying that the psyche is more individual?

LUCIA: Well, that's the way I look at it.

MARIA: Kay, you were saying that Neumann and Kalff's theory puts the manifestation of the Self at two or three years of age, but I think the Self is there from birth.

LUCIA: The Self is there all the time.

MARIA: It *appears* in a child's first drawings as a circle at around two or three when children become conscious of their own experience.

KAY: This to me is the manifestation of the Self. And is the manifestation of the Self and the constellation of the Self the same thing?

LUCIA: Yes, I don't know the difference.

MARIA: I don't make that differentiation. The manifestation of the Self is something that the individual can relate to, whether it's done in a drawing or sandplay. The imagination is the part of us that is able to imagine something that we know nothing about and then we can imagine what that might be. And so the Self takes all these different forms that we created, and a god or a goddess is one of the many forms the manifestation of the Self may take.

LUCIA: At about the age of two or three or four, children begin to be able to – image or express the Self, but what if it's there all the time?

MARIA: I think it is. At the beginning, from birth onwards, the experience of the Self is a body experience. It's a somatic experience. The experience of imagination and of Self is in the body. Fordham describes it this way.

LUCIA: Imagination is in the body – when the child is born?

MARIA: It comes through the body. The baby imagines the breast of the mother; the breast is something the baby is programmed to know. It's not as if it comes out of nowhere. There's something in the baby that knows.

KAY: That's interesting.

MARIA: The baby knows breast. It knows mouth on breast.

KAY: It's instinct?

MARIA: Yeah, it's instinct that is connected to imagination. Instinct, to me, and imagination are experienced together, especially in those early months. They're not separate.

LUCIA: I think of imagination as something that I have not experienced – directly. So I create an image of something that could possibly be, but I haven't experienced it. When I've experienced something, there's no imagination about it. I know what it is.

MARIA: Okay, if you take that definition which I think is a good one, you could apply it to a baby before it goes to the breast. It knows it's hungry. It feels hunger. And then I suppose that there's some knowledge that something will satisfy that hunger, and the breast is what the baby imagines even though it doesn't know what breast is.

LUCIA: Yes. And if you put something else to the baby's mouth that is not a breast, it sucks.

MARIA: So it knows something about sucking.

LUCIA: The sucking reflexes are present.

MARIA: Right. So there's something there about instinct.

LUCIA: Okay.

MARIA: But then it does get a breast, and then there's a whole beginning imagination about what the breast is. If the breast is there it becomes good and if it is not there it becomes bad. This is the beginning of fantasy and then imagination according to Klein and Winnicott.

KAY: See? This is where we get back to theory again.

MARIA: So the breast is actually there, but we fantasize and then imagine about breast and our inner life emerges from these experiences. Why then does the breast appear in the tray later? What the breast is, is part of our imaginal world.

KAY: I wonder if the breast appears in trays of sandplayers that have been raised on bottles only.

MARIA: It certainly did in my trays and I was raised on the bottle.

KAY: Oh, from birth?

MARIA: Yeah.

KAY: You never had a breast?

MARIA: Never had a breast.

KAY: So, since we have an n of one, this means that all 100 percent of our subjects who were raised on a bottle have had images of breasts in the tray. That's what people do with research.

MARIA: Well, we don't need to get hung up on the definitions of imagination; if the Self is something we don't know, then the only thing we can do is imagine about it.

LUCIA: And try to define it. Yeah.

KAY: And theorize about it. So someone comes along and has a big following and they theorize about these things and then we go along with that for a while, and then someone else comes along and – a new theory . . .

LUCIA: But that *is* imagination.

MARIA: Theory is imagination. Color, size, and quantity are imaginal concepts and are part of the imagination.

LUCIA: Yes.

KAY: But the imagination about theory is not universal, and imagination about the breast is universal. So that's a big difference.

MARIA: Yes.

LUCIA: And imagination about Self, or God, is universal.

KAY: Except the gods change a lot.

MARIA: It's cultural and universal.

LUCIA: It's cultural but it is part of an imaginative process. So the imagination is culturally defined but it's very important to validate the imagination, especially in describing the indescribable. It's very important for you to let me imagine Self and not tell me, "No, that's not Self. This is Self."

MARIA: And that's what's so beautiful about sandplay. It gives people the space to imagine the most unimaginable.

LUCIA: Yes, and we, as sandplay therapists, know, "That's perfect. That's exactly right."

KAY: And we aren't using words. We don't have to use words and they don't either; they just use the sand, water and objects. It seems so simple. We don't have to define the word "Self."

LUCIA: Isn't that lovely?

MARIA: Yeah. And what is so wonderful is that you, as the therapist, have an experience of the Self along with the sandplayers when *they* create it.

KAY: From the feeling in myself and the feeling between us. I, too, have a Self that I experience.

MARIA: And the sandplayer needs that reflected back: that you know, with them, that this *something happened*.

LUCIA: Absolutely.

KAY: I know that they know, that I know, that they know that I know.

MARIA: Yes, exactly, and that *this* is what we're both experiencing.

KAY: And that is very, very healing.

LUCIA: Yes.

MARIA: And essential. And *that* is what I couldn't get out of verbal therapy.

LUCIA: Do you remember when Dora showed the Self trays? In viewing the Self trays, you could not say, okay, that's it. It was that one *and* that one *and* that one *and* that one *and* that one. So the infinity of imagination around something like the Self is – is an awesome thing. It has richness and depth.

KAY: It's creative, it's healing and you really feel great.

LUCIA: Oh! Even though you didn't make one of those sand pictures, you saw it and you resonated with every single one.

MARIA: I wrote up the case of this girl who made a Self drawing, and she said at the end, "I want you to sign this." And I looked at her and I said, "I didn't make this. You made that drawing. You drew that drawing." And she said – she put her hands on her hips in this adolescent way and said, "What do you mean you didn't make it? Do you think I could have made that without you?"

KAY: That's lovely.

LUCIA: That's it right there.

MARIA: So I had to sign it with her.

LUCIA: And that's the mother. If the mother is present, then it happens. Dora Kalff said that around age three, children have an imaginal experience of the Self – a consciousness of Self created by the imagination.

KAY: Dora called it a constellation. If it doesn't occur at that time, then it may occur later in therapy. Dora said that in sandplay therapy the Self can appear. It's the mother–child unity that allows it to come.

LUCIA: And it's the same thing that your nine-year-old girl felt when she did that drawing. Without you, she couldn't have done it. In other words, she couldn't have imagined a form to put on that paper.

MARIA: Well, she couldn't have an experience of the Self that –

LUCIA: That would have allowed her to imagine –

MARIA: To imagine and then draw it.

KAY: Yeah. Imagine and experience are kind of close, aren't they? Whatever you put in the tray, you imagine and image it. Then you put it in the tray, and then that allows you to experience it. It is better than just having it in your head.

LUCIA: That's true.

KAY: That's why it's the doing of the tray that's healing, not the analysis of it.

MARIA: Yes, I agree. I was just thinking about this other little girl that I'm working with who had a very good mother connection early on, but she's an only child and she's the center of her parents' world. The presenting problem is anger and hitting her mother. She's trying to separate, have her own separate existence but she's in this nice, good uroboric oneness with the mother that she's not able to get out of. She does these beautiful trays, for instance the one with a little duck and a baby duck in a pond or a beautiful nature scene with animals and babies and then at the end, she'll stick in a volcano. She has to blow out that uroboric oneness because she's trying to develop.

KAY: The mother needs uroboric oneness. The mother–child unity has to come first but then there has to be a time when the mother can allow the separation.

MARIA: So that the separation out of the Self can happen and the child can develop and individuate.

LUCIA: So that they know that the Self is not Mother. Mother does not own the Self and your girl's mother owns her daughter's Self and that's devouring. It's a terrible thing.

MARIA: Yes, it is. It makes me think about Joseph Henderson's identification of two aspects of the Self in *Shadow and Self*: the primal Self, which is that early uroboric oneness with the mother, and the ultimate Self, which is the transcendent, spiritual Self. And that's oneness with the universe.

KAY: That is a good differentiation.

MARIA: I find that differentiation very helpful when looking at trays because you can sometimes see the Self as this uroboric oneness and other times it has a more transcendent quality to it. The ultimate Self is like the *unus mundus*, which Jung writes about in *Mysterium Coniunctionis*. In this experience of the ultimate Self, one is connected or united with the whole world, not just united with mother.

LUCIA: That's individuation, isn't it, going from the primal Self to the ultimate Self?

KAY: But you don't lose the primal Self. Don't you get to a place where you can include both, the primal Self and the ultimate Self? This seems to make sense.

MARIA: I would think so. And then what is the role of the anima and the animus in that process?

LUCIA: In the individuation process?

KAY: Well, it seems to me as though the anima, the feminine – in either man or woman – is operating for the primal Self and the masculine, or the animus, is operating for the ultimate Self.

MARIA: So maybe the feminine is the connecting link for both men and women to the primal unity and the masculine is the connecting link for women and men to the ultimate Self.

KAY: I've never seen this or thought about this before but I think it's kind of interesting.

LUCIA: All of the masculine and all of the feminine energies are present as well as a lot of other things within us, and the Self knows or is it the psyche that knows? Something knows what needs to be encouraged and developed and healed and will direct that individual, consciously or unconsciously, most of the time, to the place where that undeveloped part can be brought forth.

KAY: Good. Both Jung and Dora talk about the psyche as knowing the healing direction and being the totality that reaches for wholeness. The psyche guides the self-healing.

MARIA: So the psyche is what reaches for self-healing?

KAY: And when the Self is experienced, then the two are working together. And psyche and Self are less differentiated.

LUCIA: That's true. Yeah. I like that a lot. So the psyche then becomes more Self-like.

KAY: The two, psyche and Self, get together, because at first it's the psyche that pushes toward individuation.

MARIA: Great. And then they're working together in an interconnected way. The circumference of a circle and the center of the circle – that is all the Self, and it includes the psyche.

KAY: And the Self is the center?

MARIA: But the Self is both the center of the circle and the circumference of the circle and the psyche is the area in between. I think that's how I understand it.

LUCIA: Now, if what we have expressed about the Self being experienced early on if the holding is there is true, then the psyche knows the Self. The psyche has had that experience of the Self and knows that it can have another. So that initial experience is essential.

KAY: Okay.

LUCIA: It provides the path. Earlier, I said something about the call. I hear the call of the Self and I want to experience it again because I already have experienced it, maybe, at three. And I'm seeking it – the psyche is always seeking that experience. And that's what pulls us onward, I think, in the individuation process. Now, children who have not experienced that don't have that sense of wholeness at all. Their experience is just fractured –

MARIA: And chaotic. So many children are damaged in this way.

LUCIA: And there is an awareness by the therapists who work with these children that they can never be whole when they reach ten, eleven, twelve without having had an experience of the Self.

MARIA: No. I think there's always the potential for healing. I am always surprised at the resiliency in some of the most damaged children.

LUCIA: But the damage is so profoundly ingrained at that point in time. So that early – early experience of the Self is the call for the rest of our lives even though we don't know it. Even though we never imagined it.

KAY: 'Cause it's unconscious.

MARIA: Well, I think that's what the whole attachment theory is trying to get at, by focusing on the necessary environmental conditions needed for providing a space for this primal unity of the Self to happen. They don't talk about the Self but that's what attachment theory is all about.

LUCIA: That's right.

MARIA: It's about providing a space for the psyche to congeal in a way that an experience of the Self through relationship can happen whether it is early on in development or later in therapy.

KAY: And that's an experience that is not possible to say in words. In some therapies there is a tendency to pull things apart. In sandplay we think about putting things together. We just stay there – stay with this person, give them the experience of the mother–child unity, without our pulling things apart.

MARIA: So then one could have that experience of unity in the sand even if one hasn't had this experience of unity early on.

KAY: Right. I don't like the pulling apart.

MARIA: Well, that's not enough.

KAY: What – the pulling apart?

MARIA: My own experience in analysis was that the verbal pulling apart was not enough. I needed a nonverbal experience of the Self and I needed it affirmed in the sandplay. It was not enough for me to just talk about my experiences or my dreams; it was also important to have the experience of the Self in the sandplay so that I could hold on to the good.

LUCIA: That's right. I'm thinking of the Rider Tarot card, the Hermit. It's an image of one individual alone, carrying a lantern and trying to find the way. The interesting thing about it is that we have the lantern and we're lighting our own way. We're lighting our *own way!* No one *else* is holding it. *We* are holding the light.

KAY: We, meaning the psyche? The Self?

MARIA: Or the person who's going on the journey?

LUCIA: If we have that experience of the light, we will carry it and light our own way. I don't think there's any question about that.

MARIA: Well, I have to amend that image of the Hermit, if you are referring to sandplay. I think you have to have somebody in the background who's holding the space. In that image, there are hands around the top of the Hermit card. There needs to be the containing from the Self that is held by the therapist so that sandplayers can find their own way.

LUCIA: Well I was talking about the whole life with a little holding along the way. Mm?

KAY: I often see people who have to have some experience of the Self or a light at the end of the tunnel, in order to get through all the pain to get there. They can't just – just go on and not know that there's anything there. So they put a Self-object into the tray – a jewel or something – that they can experience and hold onto. It isn't the whole experience of the Self yet but it goes with them.

LUCIA: Exactly.

KAY: There has to be an inkling that the Self is there, and then you can go on and tolerate the pain that comes with getting there. It's hard to keep going without knowing that there's something there.

LUCIA: That's right.

KAY: And you can't be told it.

MARIA: Right. In the sand, you can actually see, feel, and experience the Self-constellation. The person gets enough strength and grounded-ness in that place that then they can face the most horrific things in the sand.

KAY: Yes. But you know you have to almost have the chaos first and the hurt first. You have to hurt enough so that something in you shows you that there is this – this Self – that you can go to. You go back and forth. You go from chaos, then you see this light. Then you get chaos again.

LUCIA: Right. And the little object is there each time.

KAY: It may be a different object each time one creates a sandtray. But there's a Self-object. And there is a difference between a Self tray and a Self-object in the tray.

MARIA: You call it a Self-object, meaning capital "S" Self-object?

KAY: Yes.

MARIA: And I think that's right. The Self-object can be a treasure or some-times a flower or a jewel.

KAY: Mm-hmm. And then you know that the sandplayer is in process and can do it.

MARIA: Yes. That is helpful.

KAY: We are seeing little Self representations within a tray, before we get to the Self trays.

LUCIA: We're back to where we started, which is that the Self – whatever that is – is there all the time.

KAY: Because, otherwise, you wouldn't have a Self-object.

LUCIA: That's right.

KAY: You couldn't.

LUCIA: It's there all the time. And our experience of it comes intermittently and we seek it, but we don't develop it because it's there. It's just there.

KAY: Then what's the difference between a Self-object and a Self tray? I guess the difference between a Self-object and Self tray is that with a Self tray you finally get to a sense of wholeness, whereas the Self-object is just telling you that the Self is there.

LUCIA: I think the Self-object is like a little – teeny little companion – that keeps your hope going. Then you can go through all that chaos and all that mess.

MARIA: And then you can go down and do it all again.

Chapter 18

Self

Maria Ellen Chiaia

> In the last resort every genuine encounter between two human beings must be conceived of as *mysterium coniunctionis*. The living mystery of life is always hidden between Two, and it is the true mystery which cannot be betrayed by words and depleted by arguments.
>
> (Jung, 1979, p. 125)

In the sandplay work I will present in this chapter, the therapist and the client met at the level of the Self in the co-transference. The intellectual, physical and spiritual development of a young woman occurred in the safe place provided by sandplay within the relationship and co-transference with an older woman therapist. In the work I will be describing, a young woman I'll call Jessica came to a sacred initiation into her own womanhood, after a meeting at the level of the Self was acknowledged between them.

I will emphasize the role of the relationship, the presence of the therapist, and the co-transference as of utmost importance in creating the free and protected space and the meeting that occurs at the level of the Self. Jungian psychology, object relations, self psychology and feminist relational theory have contributed to my thinking about what occurs in the psychotherapeutic relationship in the following case. These theoretical models emphasize the relationship between the therapist and client as a key factor in healing. I will attempt to bring the relationship into focus and discuss how the co-transference relationship is key to the appearance of the Self followed by a meeting at the level of the Self. In this case an acknowledgment of a meeting at the level of the Self was essential.

"Jessica" began therapy at the age of nine. I will be reporting her development through the age of fourteen, focusing on what occurred during the year when she was thirteen years old. Jessica started therapy because of a learning disability, having just been held back one grade in school. When she came to me, she was in emotional turmoil.

The connection and attachment between Jessica and me was mysterious and healing. She was, like me, of Italian-American descent and she looked as if she could be my daughter. The colorings of our skin, hair and eyes were similar. These similarities contributed to my identification with and understanding of Jessica, which evoked a mother–daughter co-transference. In working with Jessica I was aware of the possible negative implications of this positive co-transference: over-identification; avoidance of the negative transference including feelings of anger, envy, and hate. However, in retrospect it can be seen that her individual, personal self-development was to occur within and from the positive identification. In one of our first sessions, Jessica created a sculpture of two figures and a baby. She said, "This is you and me, and our baby." This sculpture could represent a new Self arising out of the Great Mother archetype that had been constellated (Signell, 1991, pp. 49–65).

I will discuss the events and symbolic material that led up to and followed the beginning of Jessica's menses. I would like to propose that her participation in the process that unfolded was presaged, reflected and constellated in her work with drawings and sandplay.

When Jessica was thirteen and in the fourth year of therapy, she began a session telling me about her anger and frustration at her family, particularly her brother and her sister. She was worrying about their behavior. Her older brother smoked too much pot, and her older sister spent too much time away from home. Jessica was upset because she couldn't change them. Then she spoke of her anger and frustration at our world. "How can I have children and bring them into this world when we are destroying it?" she said. She spoke of the destruction of the rainforests, all the endangered animals, the pollution of our environment and the disappearance of our trees.

Then, in response to the question Jessica posed above, about bringing children into the world, I asked her if she wanted to do a drawing. She produced a mandala-like picture. She described the drawing as follows:

> In the center is the black and red. This is me. The swirling circles in green and pink are my worries and insecurities. The next colored circles are an ozone layer, which is protecting me. And then, the lightning bolts are coming in as energy to expand and open me up. I'll never have one answer but at least I'm free to have the questions.

She called this piece Sacred Wonders.

In studying this picture as if it were a tray (Figure 18.1), I am aware of three concentric circles in the center, possibly representing the three levels of Jessica's unconscious psyche. Jessica identified the inner circle as herself.

The center holds a tension of opposites, red and black, held within a circle, like the Chinese yin–yang symbol. Cooper states, "The yin–yang symbol, the *Ta ki*, depicts the perfect balance of the two great forces . . . complementary opposites in the dualistic universe" (1988, p. 196). Cooper equates black with the yin principle. It is the darkest color, and it swallows up all the others, like death. In European countries, black is the color worn in mourning to honor

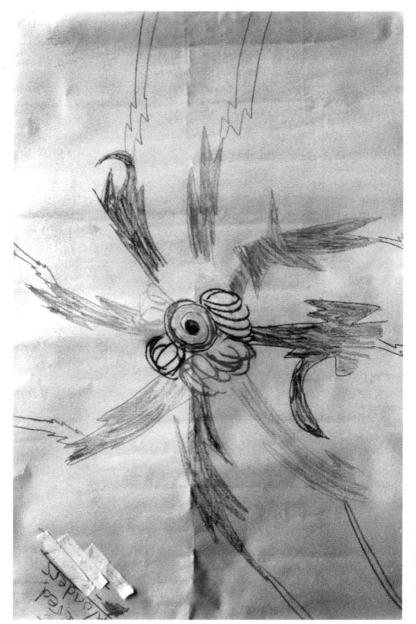

Figure 18.1 A tray by Jessica

the dead. Red is the color of blood and, in this case possibly the coming menstrual blood, which is the beginning of a girl's ability to create life. Neumann equates blood (red) with life (1964, p. 55). So in the center of this drawing, we behold life and death held in a delicate balance.

The next circle seems to represent the personal unconscious, all of Jessica's "worries and insecurities," the place where Jessica's individual, family and cultural complexes resided. The colors of this spiral, which take Jessica clockwise out into the world, are lavender and light green. Cirlot states that "secondary or tertiary colours will express symbols of more complexity" (1982, pp. 54–55). Certainly an adolescent's relationships to her family, friends and the world around her are complex, and the struggle to understand the complexity may be confusing. Jessica seemed to have begun asking philosophical and spiritual questions about life and power, about the survival of the plants and animals of the earth: questions concerning life and death. The beginning of her own menses would take her right to the center of this dilemma, as she would then have the ability to create life each month.

The third circular layer she called the ozone, which is interesting because this is the atmospheric layer that protects the earth's atmosphere. The ozone surrounds, contains and protects all life on this planet, and yet it is unseen, unknowable through our senses. For this layer Jessica used the first four colors, plus two new ones, pink and blue. This suggested to me that she included all that is known to her up to this point, plus something else. I imagine she was attempting to protect and contain the totality of her conscious and unconscious life.

And finally, she put eight lightning bolts in red, black and blue that broke into the drawing from the outside world. Cirlot writes that the lightning bolt "expresses the action of the higher [world] on the lower . . . it is an active force, terrible and dynamic" (1982, p. 342). As an adolescent, Jessica faced many of life's challenges, tests and difficulties. She had traveled through life and faced many developmental tasks. She said that those were lightning bolts coming in; I saw the lightning bolts as energy coming in and expanding her.

Let us look at the eight lightning bolts in another way. The number eight is four doubled, a double quaternio. In *Mysterium Coniunctionis* there is a diagram showing a similar double quaternio pattern. Jung says, "The double quaternio or ogdoad stands for a totality, for something that is at once heavenly and earthly, spiritual or corporeal, and is found in the . . . unconscious" (1963, par. 8). So, the whole drawing is an expression of the totality of the Self. If the drawing was preparing Jessica, on the psychological and spiritual level, for the coming of menses on the corporeal level, then the appearance of the Self is essential. Kalff writes, "a healthy development of the ego can only take place as a result of the successful manifestation of the Self. Such a manifestation of the Self seems to guarantee the development and consolidation of the personality" (1980, p. 29).

After Jessica completed the drawing, there was an unspoken feeling of mystery and sacredness in the room. As mentioned above, she called this picture Sacred Wonders. Jessica then signed the drawing and asked me to sign it too. I said, "But Jessica, I didn't make it. You made the drawing." She looked at me with a puzzled expression and replied, "I couldn't have done this without you. We've created this together." I think she was referring to the four years of therapy and remembering and honoring the relationship that had developed in the co-transference in order for this meeting at the level of the Self to occur.

I thanked her for reminding me, and silently remembered that out of deep relationship the numinous can arise and that the Self, or the living mystery of life as Jung said, is always found in an "other." I created the free and protected space; Jessica drew the picture; Jessica created the expression of the Self. When she stated that we created the drawing together, I was filled with a sense of the presence of the divine and I knew that Jessica and I had met at the level of the Self.

I wondered if Jessica's expressed desire – her wanting me to sign the drawing with her in recognition of a connection and meeting – was the beginning of a modern-day puberty rite. Because of the quality of feeling that emerged between us, I wondered if, in the above events, both symbolic and instinctual archetypes were activated and a puberty rite was set in motion by her experience of a spiritual communion with me, an older woman. Did the drawing of the picture, the asking me to sign it, and the quality of the feelings that emerged, all contribute to this movement within her psyche?

From January to September, for nine months following the drawing, Jessica would arrive at the sessions relieved that she had a private place to discuss and integrate the dynamic forces that were breaking in (the lightning bolts). She seemed preoccupied with having a developing new body, new feelings and new sensations, and she talked about the difficulties that arose from her encounter with the world in her new form. Most of the time I just listened, mirroring her thoughts and feelings back to her, so she could begin to know the young woman she was becoming.

About nine months later, when she had just turned fourteen, Jessica arrived in an excited state. "Guess what happened last week?" she asked. "Can you give me some clues?" I replied. "Well, it's happening right now!" she exclaimed. I was puzzled for a few moments and then it came to me. "You got your period!" "Yes," she cried. "And it started last week right here in your office." I was awed by this occurrence. There were no words, only a silence filled with meaning and deep connection.

Again, as I reflect back on the above events, this is what occurs to me. After the making of Sacred Wonders, Jessica withdrew from doing any sandplay and drawings for nine months, the amount of time needed for a pregnancy. Perhaps what was occurring was a psychological pregnancy, and then menstruation began. It was as if there had been a psychic union, a psychological pregnancy, and then the birth of a young woman into womanhood in my presence. This felt like a holy mystery of life "hidden between Two" (Jung, 1979, p. 125), in this case two women, joined together in a woman's mystery. When menstruation began in my office in my presence, there was in that moment the coming together of the individual, the relationship, the biological, the collective, and the archetypal. And this is where the mystery is. Together we participated in the mystery, and, again, we met at the level of the Self, this time biologically. Of course, none of this was interpreted to her, yet there was an unspoken feeling of this mystery held between us.

Returning to the session, after a long silence, she exclaimed, "I am bleeding now, a drop just fell." We laughed together. She told me how important it was to see *her* blood in her bed, on her white sheets. *Her* blood now, not her mother's or her sister's. She told me how she walked around her room naked and rejoiced when her blood stained the floor. Again she said excitedly, "A drop just fell, right now."

Then I asked her what it meant to her to have her period. She said, "I am a woman. I am in the cycle of life. I am part of the feminine crowd. Each drop of blood that comes from me reminds me of my responsibility towards my body and possible children I may have."

Jessica spoke of a highly individual experience of *her* blood and yet her entrance into the "cycle of life and the feminine crowd," which is a collective, archetypal experience. We met at the level of the Self; she merged with the continuity of the feminine, and yet was differentiated from her mother, her sister and me. I think my nonverbal holding of this understanding made possible what followed.

Coming back to the session, Jessica then asked to do a sandtray. Jessica worked with sandtray figures of the Great Mother (Figure 18.2).

Jessica began by really working the sand, which showed her deep involvement. She purposefully placed twelve goddesses in a semicircle around the tray. She put Shiva in the top center. The twelve goddesses from left to right are a sorcerer/shaman I call Morgaine, the Virgin Mary, an early (3000 BC) earth goddess, the Virgin, Shiva, another Virgin, a snake goddess from Crete, the Madonna (Virgin and Child), another Madonna, an angel, the Virgin, and the Venus of Willendorf. In the front center, she made a pool of water and placed a crystal ball in the middle of the water. Around the pool, she placed six animals: a seal, three frogs (one with a baby on its back), and two turtles (one with a baby on its back).

As in the drawing, Jessica again assembled two concentric circles; in the outer is a panoply of feminine goddesses with Shiva (God of creation and destruction) in the middle, and then there is an inner circle of animals. She said they had all "come . . . to watch the power source of love and tranquility." In the center of the large pool of water is the crystal ball, which she called the power source.

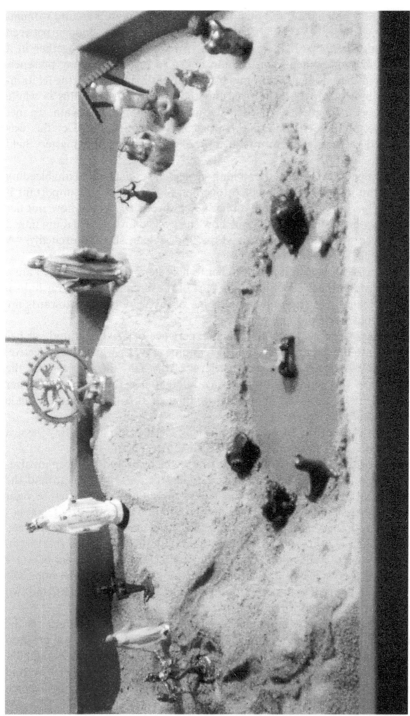

Figure 18.2 A tray by Jessica

In each of the goddesses, there is a different experience of the feminine archetype. This rite included Jessica reestablishing "contact with the world of the Gods in all their special aspects" (Eliade, 1976, p. 166).

The Virgins without children could represent women, an unmarried bride of God "belonging to herself alone, being her own mistress," which is the original meaning of the word "virgin." Virgins with children allude to the reproductive mystery that is now possible for Jessica to participate in, by giving birth not only biologically but also symbolically. Walker called the Virgin a "soul-mother" (1983, p. 1049).

These spiritual, Catholic figures alternate with physical, erotic figures. Jessica needed to know both sides of the feminine. The Venus of Willendorf is an earth, fertility goddess of the elemental kind. She shows the fullness of the feminine form in an erotic way, life-giving and not shameful. She is an early earth goddess in harmony with the elemental forces of the natural world. The snake goddess and the shaman are both transformer goddesses, holding the mystery of transformation of blood into child and into milk, as well as other transformation mysteries (Neumann, 1963). The snake goddess is also very physical and erotic, holding the phallic snake, possibly symbolic of the sexual forces about to break into Jessica's consciousness. Finally, I think of the angel as a divine messenger, a necessary presence in this rite of passage.

The animals Jessica chose live both in the water and on land. They are possibly symbolic of her instinctual potential to negotiate successfully between the inner and outer, conscious and unconscious, personal sexuality (instincts) and spirituality. And of course there are the mother and child pairs, perhaps honoring the power and magic of creation.

The following is the story she told me about the tray.

> The animals are coming from the ocean to watch the power source [she pointed to the crystal ball], which is a source of love and tranquility. These goddesses are the highest forms of spirit in the world. They too are coming, some of them with their children, to look at the power source. It is there to help them and they are there to help it. They know it but they don't know it. They know it but they don't consciously know it. The animals are there because of nature. The goddesses made them. Since they are connected to the goddesses, they get to see the power source.

At the onset of menses, within the temenos of a human relationship between two females, we get a fleeting glimpse of the emergence of a knowing of spiritual truth and power for one young woman. "But we know it and we don't know it." Henderson clearly and beautifully describes women's initiation. "What she needs . . . is the feeling of being contained in a meaningful relationship to a person who can carry the sense of its being a transcendent, not just an ordinary, experience of relationship" (1967, p. 121).

Jessica reminded me of this by having me sign the drawing. And then there was the feeling and awareness of the sacredness in the room as we met at the level of the Self. Finally, we were both surprised by the beginning of menstruation in my office. The container of therapy, the relationship to another woman, and the holding the mystery of the meeting, provided the space for an initiation to occur and for Jessica to experience the sacredness of her menstruation.

In describing these events, I hope I have shown that a meeting at the level of the Self occurred between therapist and client. Understanding this event leads to an expanded theoretical construct of the experience of the Self which includes its occurrence in the co-transference. An understanding of this occurrence is important to sandplay work.

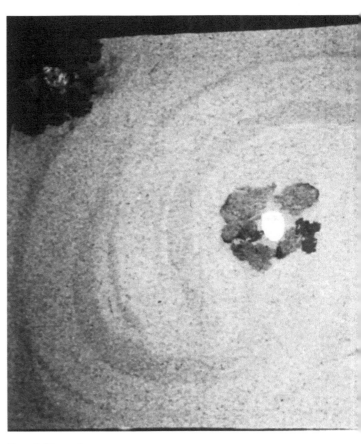

Plate 1 Therapist

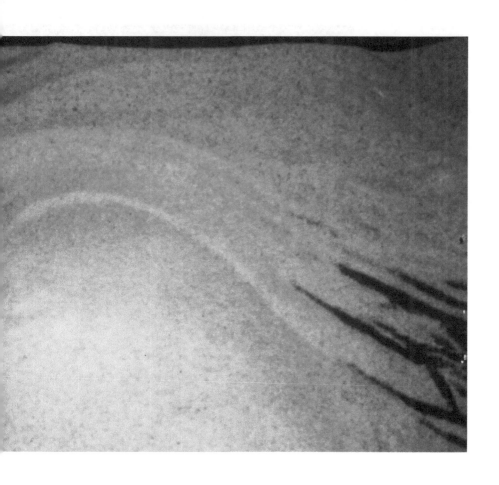

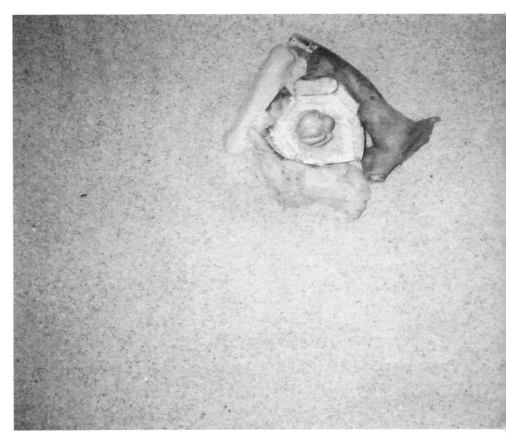

Plate 3 Child

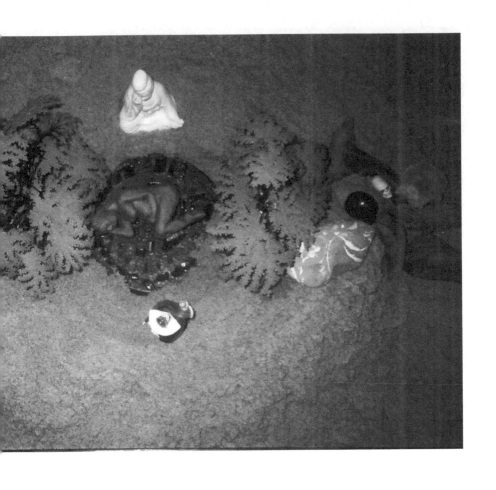

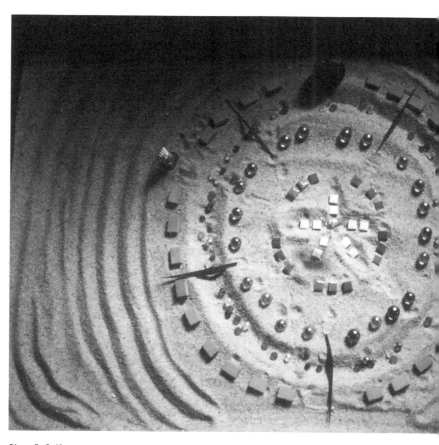

Plate 5 Self

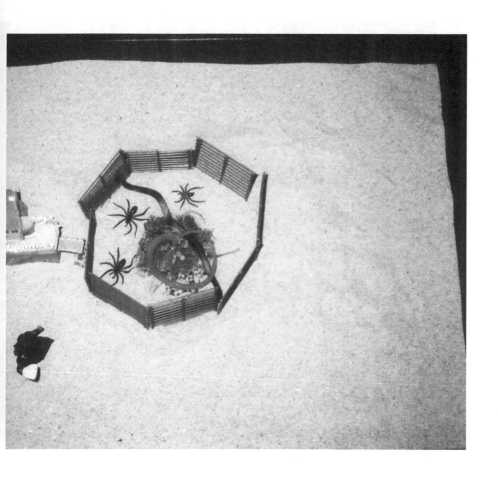

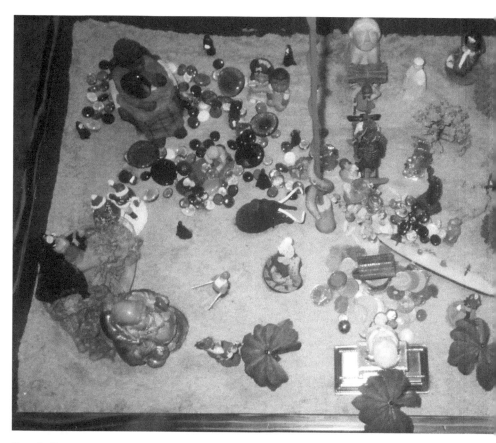

Plate 7 Chaos

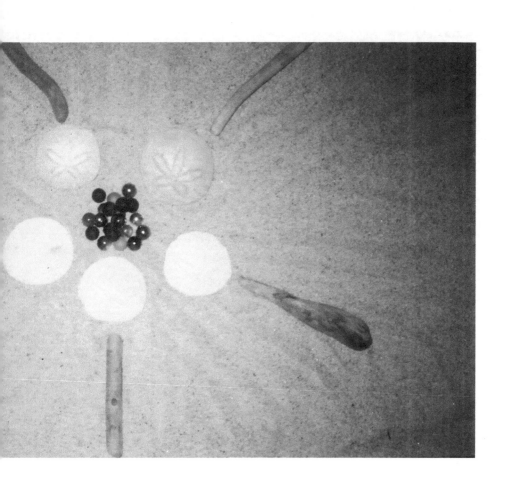

Chapter 19

Self

Kay Bradway

Depth therapies have in common a reliance on something above, below, beyond the ego that is responsible for and directs the self-healing and emotional and spiritual growth in humans. Sigmund Freud laid the groundwork with the recognition of the unconscious. C.G. Jung went further with the positing of the universal unconscious. This led to Jung's defining the archetypes which are in the universal unconscious and are recognized through symbols. He identified the central archetype as the Self, spelled with a capital "S." Since then there has been the question of "Just what is the Self?"

The "Self" has been described and defined in numerous ways by numerous analysts. It has universally been seen as powerful in its relation to the ego.

John Beebe has pointed out that Jung saw the Self as having the ability "to cancel our wishes, frustrate our wills, and intensify our fears all in the service of a mysterious project: Individuation" (2003).

Jungian analysts find images of the Self in dreams. Sandplay therapists have thought that sandplay provided a visual method of identifying the presence of the Self. They have found that, coincidental with the apparent experiencing of the Self by the sandplayer, the sandplay scene has shown a recognizable pattern. Early on, it was thought that mandalas appeared as such a recognizable pattern. Sandplay therapists started to speak of "Self trays." But there has been lack of agreement regarding the identification of Self trays in sandplay processes. If they do exist, what are they? What do they look like? How does one recognize a Self tray? In my work with Dora Kalff, I recall her identifying some trays as "Self trays." But it has been pointed out that she did not refer to them in any of her writings. When asked about them in a public lecture, I remember Dora's saying that each one is unique, and that you cannot make any generalities about them. But then she added that they all do have one thing in common – they all are numinous; they all elicit a feeling of numinosity in the viewer. I recall when Dora Kalff presented her collection of sandplay Self scenes in a paper entitled "Beyond the Shadow" at the International Association of Analytical Psychology Conference in Berlin in 1986. At each appearance of a sandplay Self scene on the screen, there was a unanimity of "ahs" from the audience. The scenes were very different from each other, but all were numinous. All elicited that feeling of – what is it? Awe? I recall one analyst's feeling reaction on seeing the trays of her analysand for the first time at our joint viewing of the sandplay process. When we reached such a tray she whispered, "It sends goose bumps up and down my back."

However, the level of disagreement among senior sandplay therapists about the identity of Self trays, or even about the validity of their existence, prompted Scott Cameron to choose the topic "Recognizing the appearance of the Self in sandplay therapy" for his doctoral dissertation at the California School of Professional Psychology (2001).

Cameron did depth interviews with eleven senior members of Sandplay Therapists of America. He started with three primary questions.

1   What does the appearance of the Self mean with regard to sandplay therapy?
2   What are the issues related to recognizing the Self in sandplay therapy?
3   To what degree is the term "Self tray" accepted and used to refer to the sandtray that is associated with appearance of the Self in sandplay therapy?

Secondary questions were designed to answer the primary questions and included: references to recognition and meaning of the appearance of the Self; Self symbols and images of the Self; relation of the terms "manifestation" and "constellation" of the Self to the appearance of the Self; relation of the co-transference to the appearance of the Self; and the relation of sandplayers' internal experiences to their life context.

Application of sophisticated programs of statistical analysis allowed Cameron to reach significant conclusions, some of which can be paraphrased as follows.

- When the Self appears, there is a coalescence and a release of energy within the sandplayer.
- Accessing the Self becomes easier over time as the ego–Self relationship is made more conscious and developed.
- The Self is present and guiding the sandplayer's development and the sandplay process even when it is not clearly evident.
- The most reliable way to recognize the appearance of the Self is by feeling and sensing the numinous energy, which may be described as "palpable," that is present in the session when the Self is accessed.

The relationship between the sandplay therapist and sandplayer is the most important determinant related to the appearance of the Self in sandplay therapy. Whether or not the Self appears in sandplay therapy depends mainly on the quality of the therapeutic relationship. The sandplay therapist, by being empathically attuned to the sandplayer, can recognize milestones in sandplay processes including the appearance of the Self.

The Self experience is not the goal nor the end of sandplay therapy. Continued therapeutic work is required following the appearance of the Self to integrate the experience.

Chapter 20

Self

Lucia Chambers

> Intellectually the Self is no more than a psychological concept, a construct that serves to express an unknowable essence which we cannot grasp as such, since by definition it transcends our powers of comprehension. It might equally be called the "god within us."
>
> (Jung, 1966a, par. 399)

Even though Jung declared the Self to be beyond our ability to define and understand, he continued to search for a way to articulate the "knowing" within his own psyche of a powerful force. His search led him back in history to the time when image and fantasy were still an acceptable way of looking at the world, when the subjective experience was credible. In alchemy, he found "unrevealed ancient wisdom" (Corbett, 1996, p. 78). In it he discovered a metaphor for his theory of transformation and the role of the Self. In this symbolic and complicated art, a substance holding two disparate elements is placed in a sealed container. Heat is applied along with a specific series of complex procedures. The original substance is transformed and has revealed its true nature.

From a psychological perspective, the work of the ego is to identify and define us as individuals, to "materialize" as distinctly as possible. In doing so, paradoxically, the ego loses or forgets the connections with its original totality, the Self. Life becomes an experience of fragmentation, barrenness and emptiness. In order to experience the transformative processes of the alchemist, we need the courage to set out on the dangerous quest for the "gold" lost in the base matter of physical reality, the "lead." Alchemical images tell of dismemberment, burning, and torture. Some alchemists deeply involved in the process died or went mad as they quested. At the end of the process, there is a meeting of the "gross lead" of the ego and the transcendent light of the totality, or the Self. That meeting place, the third area, is where there is a union of the opposites of matter and spirit, the *coniunctio*. The conscious mind, in meeting and recognizing the "gold," is transformed and a new personality emerges, composed of both. "God is now to be carried experientially by the individual" (Corbett, 1996, p. 130).

Jung found yet another field that dealt with the process of transformation. In the Gnostic tradition, the creator becomes lost when he *creates* matter. Just by being himself, he destroys himself. His creations are the splintered remnants of himself. They wander through the world of destiny, birth and death, seeking only to escape their chaos and pain. In Gnosticism, creation seems to have been a great mistake that should not have happened. Reality seems evil. Yet the real evil is to refuse to acknowledge the splintered bits of the divine within. If awareness or the "knowing" of the divine is claimed, each bit will be moved back toward reunion with the godhead and God will be recreated.

Jung used the Gnostic metaphor to show that the ego has the responsibility for reassembling the Self, which has been fragmented and projected onto the world. The ego must realign itself with that divine source as well as maintaining its own identity. The ego has returned to the unconscious state (the godhead) in order to raise the level of consciousness of the Self so that the self can be followed. As our consciousness extends into the unconscious, we encounter images of God that we then transform. This process is one of continuous revelation (Corbett, 1996). Jung says, "It is not I who create myself, rather I happen to myself" (Rosen, 1996, p. 15).

Continuing to search for amplification on his understanding of the Self, Jung explored the Book of Job (1960). In this story, Job, representing the ego, takes a stand against God when God's commands are base in nature. He acknowledges God as the supreme power even as he is protesting that he is being mistreated by that God. God then removes his misfortunes. In other words, even though the ego (Job) is wounded, it still believes there is a meaning in the experience. Because of the ego's persistence, a transformation takes place that brings a greater understanding of the transpersonal nature of life and therefore an acceptance of it. An observing consciousness is needed to reflect the image of the Self back to the Self and thus initiate its transformation. The Self needs the ego and the ego needs the Self. The ego–Self axis is the foundation upon which the entire personality rests. Psychological experience indicates that there is a reciprocal relationship between consciousness and the central archetype. Initially this relationship can be experienced as adversarial, but when the autonomy of each is preserved, there exists a relationship that propels both toward greater transformation, responding to soul's desire to know itself.

It is no wonder that the complexities of Jung's thought processes, and the persistence with which he attempted to define "an unknowable essence" (1966a, par. 399), are part of a continuing discussion and lack of agreement concerning the concept of the Self. Polly Young-Eisendrath reports that "some Jungians regard the Self as equivalent to the soul or God, whereas others regard it as a principle of organization" (1997, p. 13). The views are substantially different. What is significant is that Jung's search has stimulated the investigative and creative minds of many who desire to more deeply understand and clarify the energy that lies in the core of the human psyche. This core energy fosters the evolution of the human, before birth and developmentally, beyond a purely biological organism.

The ongoing speculation has moved farther afield into other schools of psychology. Kohut's self psychology theorizes about the reflecting, empathic transference that opens the way to the self, which has a psychic system of its own with its own dynamic structure.

Fordham sees an *a priori self*, present at birth, which responds to stimuli from the environment with a cyclic process of deintegration and reintegration. Winnicott says there is no self at birth. From his object relations perspective, a core begins to develop through a recognition of otherness and differentness. For Winnicott there is a False Self similar to the persona, and a True Self, which he describes as an organ of meaning.

Most who explore the depths of the psyche agree that there is an order under the confusion, conflict and chaos. In sandplay we have an opportunity to encounter that energy. There is an evolution, so to speak, taking place in the very moment of creation when a "numinous" energy comes forth from the sand creation itself. This is the moment that illuminates the darkness within both the therapist and the client – an I–Thou experience occurs. Buber says, "God is that which flows between in an I–Thou relationship" (1958, p. 10).

Because the images springing from this place of numinosity are as varied as life itself, it is very difficult to define a "Self tray." In doing so, we immediately begin to limit and confine an infinite experience. It might be helpful, however, to take note of the attempt of Corbett (1996) to roughly group images.

1   The mandala, in Sanskrit meaning "magic circle," is one of the most easily recognized centering images appearing in the sand. A quaternary encompassed within the form of a circle of objects, composed, usually but not always, of organic materials such as rocks, wood or shells – or perhaps crystals or jewels – make the circular form.
2   A central item or items from nature or of organic origin might be present in the sand to symbolize the primal energy of the Self: flowers, fish, shells, crystals, gold, rocks, mounds, wood and bodies of water.
3   A centering figure having a religious or transcendent association might appear, such as Christ, Buddha, Tara, Kuan Yin, Shiva or figures from many mythologies.
4   A pair of opposites might appear together, such as a king and queen, a lion and a lamb, black and white, or fire and water.

We need to be especially careful of using any categorizing system to label a particular tray. When we use the intellect to identify an image, we immediately reduce an archetype into the realm of the personal, and in doing so we lose the very meaning that is held by the mystery appearing before us.

For millennia, perhaps since the beginning of the time when humankind began to be aware of an "Otherness," there has been a search for a clearer and deeper understanding of that which is part of us but not of us. Philosophers, theologians, scientists, psychologists, authors and poets have all participated in the ancient ritual of circumambulation that honors a cosmic quality, circling round and round that which holds the center.

Jung gives formal recognition to the poet. The archetypal impact of poetry:

> stirs us because it summons up a voice stronger than our own. Whoever speaks in primordial images speaks with a thousand voices ... He transmutes our personal destiny into the destiny of mankind, and evokes in us all those beneficent forces that ever and anon have enabled humanity to find a refuge from every peril and to outlive the longest night.
>
> (1966b, par. 129)

Rumi, one of the world's greatest spiritual poets, is perhaps speaking of the individuation process and of the Self when he speaks with his infinite voice:

> Work. Keep digging your well.
> Don't think about getting off from work.
> Water is there somewhere.
>
> Keep knocking, and the joy inside
> Will eventually open a window
> And look out to see who's there.
>
> Rumi

Part VI

Shadow

Chapter 21

Shadow trialogue

KAY: The first time I ever heard the word "shadow" used in a psychological way was that song "Me and My Shadow." Remember that?

ALL: [laughter]

LUCIA: That's such a sweet little song, too.

KAY: Yes. "Me and my shadow da da da da . . ." We are just walking along the avenue together and we are alone. It isn't negative at all. And then I started to hear "shadow" in the Jungian group and it was all bad. And then I heard that Jung allowed its being good and bad. So that changed my whole picture of the shadow, but it's very hard to get rid of the feeling that "shadow" is negative. But I suppose that a criminal's shadow must be positive.

LUCIA: The clinical definition of "shadow" is that it is all of the unexpressed, unwanted, unacknowledged, unrecognized parts of our personality.

MARIA: It's the unrecognized and unwanted parts of more than the personality –

KAY: Of our whole being. It contributes to the whole. And we wouldn't have a whole if we didn't have a shadow.

LUCIA: That's right.

KAY: We don't have the whole till we recognize shadow. When we get to shadow, we have to recognize both the positive and negative. And to recognize the positive helps in recognizing the negative. I mean, you aren't so afraid to face the shadow because you know both the positive and negative are part of us.

MARIA: So, for example, if somebody is identified with being depressed and unhappy and sad, then that person's shadow is actually happy and joyous.

KAY: Or even manic. That's a negative way of saying it.

MARIA: But the shadow could be that extreme. Yeah. But I think a lot of people hear "shadow" and they think "dark" and then you can get into racist ideas. "Dark" is bad. Although, for some people, the light is the shadow because they're so identified with the dark. I know this is true for me as I've struggled with depression. So light and happiness is a shadow for me.

KAY: But you have to acknowledge it and realize it's there.

MARIA: Exactly. And let it live through me.

LUCIA: If we're going to do black and white or positive and negative, then you can have a white shadow. But there we have the judgments again. When we label something either positive or negative, I think we get into trouble. The shadow is just a part that is not as conscious, or not as recognized, as another part. It isn't necessarily bad or good.

KAY: I don't think Maria has said anything about bad or good. She's saying that there's a depressive part, but she's not saying it's bad, but that it's overemphasized. And then the unconscious brings up joy and lightness to compensate.

LUCIA: I was just saying to Maria that lightness is part of her shadow which is a very interesting conversation. You see? Light in the shadow.

KAY: That's what is hard for people to accept.

LUCIA: I've had such interesting experiences living in the middle of the high tech world. Men usually only come to see me when things are *really* bad. And they often have Italian silk suits and Gucci loafers. They look perfect – perfect! And in the beginning I was totally intimidated by these men because they didn't look like they had any shadow – they were so perfect. And they were earning four times as much as I was earning.

ALL: [laughter]

LUCIA: I remember one man's saying after a few minutes of introduction, "Look at my hands." And he lifted his hands and they were shaking – just shaking. The concept of "shadow" was very helpful. I would think, "Okay. Here is this man who is totally logical, competitive, linear –"

KAY: Living out what the goal is for men.

LUCIA: Yes, what's the opposite of that? If we're going for shadow, what is the opposite of that?

MARIA: What did you think of, Lucia?

LUCIA: The spiritual being –

MARIA: Yes, the nonmaterial being.

LUCIA: One man I worked with had a five-car garage with an incredibly expensive car in every garage. I started going for the shadow 'cause he was just too perfect. And perfect is flat. Do you know?

KAY: Mm-hmm, flat and perfect.

LUCIA: Flat perfect. So we went back toward the child, when the wholeness may have been more alive. We went back until he was around fifteen. At that time this man had worked for a construction company in the summer time to earn money. And one of the construction sites was up in the mountains where he was helping to build a meditation center.

KAY: Meditation center?

LUCIA: Yeah, and when he had a break he would go and listen to the monks. And then he would sit and meditate with them. He said that was the happiest time that he could ever remember. So we talked about whether he could bring this back into his life now. This spirituality was his shadow. After months of trying to figure this out, he found a little six-foot space in the back corner of one of his five garages and fenced it off with a screen. There he put a table with a Buddha, an incense burner, a pillow and a heater. And he would sneak out there when he could. He said, "I can't let anybody know about this."

KAY: Except you.

LUCIA: Except me. And I then wondered how to help him integrate that shadow. He was not conscious of it and owning it.

MARIA: Well, not quite. He did make a little place for it in his garage, even though it was a little, tiny space and among the cars.

KAY: But it's a great step.

LUCIA: Exactly, but how will he integrate that shadow?

KAY: Well, he will do it. He's done it this far. You've given him a space, and each person does it differently. And there's no generalizing how this integration occurs. It is marvelous that he's gotten this far.

MARIA: Yes.

KAY: It's his own thing. He may not get any further in expressing it. But he's done a lot, I think.

LUCIA: Okay. But how far can you go?

KAY: You mean the therapist or the client?

LUCIA: What I mean is how far do I want them to go? I know I'm not supposed to want.

KAY: Well, you can't help it, though. All right. You admit you want.

ALL: [laughter]

MARIA: That's your shadow.

LUCIA: That is my shadow.

MARIA: Did he find his shadow in the sand?

LUCIA: No, he never did sand.

MARIA: So what about shadow in the sand? How do we identify what the shadow is?

KAY: Do we have to?

LUCIA: I think we need to be careful here. I've seen a lot of sandplay presentations, and often anything that's black or scary – a witch or a devil or even a gorilla – is seen as shadow. And what's scary is bad. To automatically identify something as negative suggests that you need to get rid of it or that it doesn't have a place.

KAY: As sandplay therapists, we're different from most people because we know it doesn't have to be gotten rid of. And our knowing this is what is healing for the sandplayer.

LUCIA: Yes. In the sand there is always a place for the dark and the scary – for witches or whatever might appear.

MARIA: And maybe what you were saying earlier, Kay, about not having to identify the shadow in the sandtray specifically, is important. Whether you identify the shadow or not, the sandplayer is experiencing being held in such a way that the shadow is accepted. And from this acceptance it will be integrated. And it *is* being integrated.

KAY: Now, in sandplay, they build something, in the sand, right? They might put in the witch.

MARIA: And the witch might not be the shadow or it might be the shadow but it really doesn't matter. By just making the sand, they've had an experience of integration.

KAY: Right. That's what I think. I think we may be developing new theories. In sandplay we don't have to stay with established theory since we have our own unique experiences from having seen so many different sandplay processes. We have developed assurance that the process will go on and take its own course. It's not from having read about it. It's trusted experience.

LUCIA: Yes.

KAY: It is picked up by a sandplayer that we are neither praising nor damning however they may use the figures. The therapist is seeing the sandplay and the sandplayer as a whole. And that's healing.

LUCIA: And when you can play out that split-off, or unacknowledged, part of yourself in the sand, then maybe you don't have to do it as much at home or at school. But you have to do it somewhere because the shadow does not go away. It is better to do it the sand. There was a program that was called *The Shadow*.

MARIA: A radio show that was called *The Shadow Knows*.

LUCIA: And what knowledge does the shadow carry – for us – and for each individual? The shadow carries something valuable.

KAY: Yes. It carries the opposites to our conscious and so it is only by integrating it that we can experience wholeness.

LUCIA: So we should welcome the shadow, shouldn't we?

KAY: Oh, yes.

MARIA: The shadow has many levels. It may be personal but it also can be cultural, and it has archetypal aspects as well.

KAY: The shadow is not a universal archetype is it – like the Self? Because it is different for each person, I guess it doesn't represent an archetype.

MARIA: Well, it does represent archetypal reality but not a universal one.

LUCIA: Or – or one particular symbol.

KAY: But "archetypal" means that it's in a lower level of the unconscious for everybody – that it's the same.

LUCIA: It might look different.

KAY: But it would be – each person's shadow is different from the other person's shadow.

LUCIA: And maybe culturally that's true also.

MARIA: I've thought about the shadow in terms of being the opposite of the persona. Then I read Joe Henderson, and in *Shadow and Self* he puts the shadow as the opposite to the Self. He says, wherever the Self is, the shadow is. So we are holding the opposites at the deepest level of the psyche.

KAY: Okay.

MARIA: You're getting it at that archetypal level but it is in relationship to whatever the symbol of the Self is for that person. Culturally we can see in the yin–yang symbol that there is the little dot of the white in the black and the black dot in the white. In this Chinese symbol, we see opposites of the other within the other.

KAY: And the complement of the other.

MARIA: And complement – in terms of the shadow/Self level.

LUCIA: So what are you saying?

MARIA: I'm just playing with ideas. I think the shadow can be the opposite of both the persona and the Self. When you're watching someone do a sandtray, you may see different aspects of shadow manifestation.

KAY: I wonder if the shadow comes first and then the persona.

LUCIA: It doesn't become the shadow until the persona begins to be formed and excludes something or some aspect. I think that a lot of that's cultural, don't you?

KAY: Well, it's archetypal, cultural and familial.

MARIA: Yes, probably the shadow in your family was different from mine.

LUCIA: Well, I'm sure . . .

ALL: [laughter]

LUCIA: Scandinavian and Italian, I'm sure of that! So does shadow then stand for the part of us that is unconscious?

KAY: I thought you said it very well before. The shadow is the part that is unacknowledged because we don't like it. If we were like your client, whose life was about computers and material things, then our shadow would be spiritual.

LUCIA: Uh-huh.

KAY: It's unacknowledged, and as soon as he can acknowledge it – as he was doing – then he approaches wholeness, and that's what individuation is.

LUCIA: So the shadow, as it becomes acknowledged, increasingly becomes a part of who we are.

KAY: We never complete our individuation. I always like James Hall's definition of individuation.

MARIA: What was that?

KAY: In his little book *Jungian Dream Interpretation*, he said that individuation is the conscious realization of one's unique psychological reality including both our strengths and weaknesses and this leads to the experience of the Self.

LUCIA: So then, as we become more and more conscious of our shadow and own more of it, then does the shadow become deeper and – how – how does that work?

MARIA: Lucia, you were saying before that perfection is one-dimensional and that, as we begin to deepen with our shadow, we are not so flat and perfect and become more dimensional. I think we deepen as individuals. If we think of a pencil or charcoal drawing, the darker the shading, the more depth to the drawing. It's more three-dimensional. We become filled out as human beings the more we can live in relationship to those parts of us that are less conscious or split off.

KAY: So as we individuate, we don't project the shadow. We don't project it onto someone else. If we acknowledge it in ourselves, we don't have to project it. Isn't that true?

LUCIA: Yes.

MARIA: Well, we might project it but we then may become aware of the shadow. We may feel that little mean, green envy and know that it's ours. We may realize then that it's not about the other.

KAY: So we don't assign it to the other person. Or we recognize that we're assigning it and then we don't hold the person responsible. We are responsible for the shadow.

LUCIA: One more time, I have to say how wonderful sandplay is because it is nonverbal. In a verbal therapy, when we try to own the shadow it can be such awful and icky stuff. It's very hard to verbally acknowledge it. Ugh! In fact, I probably won't – except in the middle of the night when I wake up and have some awful . . .

KAY: You may have had a dream.

LUCIA: I may have had a dream. But in the sand you can begin to develop a relationship with the parts of yourself that you don't know and don't acknowledge – without shame.

KAY: And you're doing it with someone you don't have to verbalize it to, but you know they also are looking at this and are not against you for it. They're accepting you so there may not be shame.

MARIA: I think the shame can be there, for the person creating the tray. If they see the shadow for the first time, they might feel shame. But then, as the therapists, we mirror back the acceptance. Then they can work with that acceptance within themselves.

LUCIA: I agree; I don't think the shadow comes out in a sandplay process until there is a trusting relationship between therapist and sandplayer, and then the risk isn't so great. So then the shadowy stuff can begin to come out in a safe place.

KAY: And the acceptance by the therapist is not just on a verbal level.

LUCIA: I agree.

KAY: It's acceptance at a much deeper level. It's that guts to guts place we have mentioned so many times before, and you don't have to really come to conscious grips with it at first. Your psyche realizes that it's being accepted by the therapist at a very deep level.

MARIA: Right, and maybe what you're saying, Lucia, is that when the person first experiences the shadow, there's no shame. But when they step out and look at the sandtray the shame might come in. Then they may look at me and look at my facial expression, to see how I'm holding that.

LUCIA: Exactly.

KAY: Not just that the therapist seems to accept what you've created but the therapist accepts you, all of you.

LUCIA: Yeah. There's a space created in which that relationship is happening. I've never had anybody do sand where they've done deep shadow work in the first tray. You have to work your way into it – until it's safe.

KAY: In fact many times what is thought of as a "good" tray has to come before a scary tray, so that one can feel good about oneself before facing up to what is thought of as negative. I found that with a woman sand-player. She wanted to do two trays each time. She had to do a first tray that she experienced as "good," and then she could do the "bad" tray.

LUCIA: One of the reasons that sandplay can go so deeply is that, from that guts to guts relationship, there isn't anything that is wrong or –

KAY: Bad.

LUCIA: Bad or shouldn't be there. That is the unspoken agreement between the therapist and the client on that level. And I don't think you can make that kind of a verbal agreement.

KAY: I agree.

MARIA: I am wondering what is it about the sandplay that allows us to feel that guts to guts acceptance?

KAY: We aren't using words so we relate at a deeper place.

LUCIA: And it's also contained.

MARIA: The image that came to me was of a child doing a drawing. I don't judge a child's drawing.

LUCIA: No.

KAY: True.

MARIA: I just look at it and I am interested in what's being expressed. So it's somehow taken out of this personal – I can't quite get at it, help me.

LUCIA: It's an expression.

MARIA: That we just take and accept?

KAY: Perhaps it's because we're dedicated to no words – or very few words. And so it's expression without words and this has to be at a deeper level, because as soon as we get words, we come out of this deep place.

MARIA: But why is the nonverbal easier? What makes us able to not get hooked the way we would if we were having a verbal interchange with someone?

KAY: You have to think what you're going to say and put it into words. And in sandplay, you can just trust what happens without having to use words.

MARIA: Okay. I see. So it's the nonverbal that allows us to drop into this deeper place, this guts to guts connection.

KAY: I think so.

LUCIA: Then, you can just be with the flow of energy – 'cause you don't cut it off with words.

KAY: If you're in a verbal therapy and the client says something, you have to think of words to respond with. In sandplay, you are trusting something deeper than words. And you get so you can really trust it and the sandplayer trusts it and then something happens.

MARIA: I like that. It just needs to be said so many times. We, as sandplay therapists, create a free and protected space, a basic level of acceptance –

KAY: In relationship.

LUCIA: And there's a flow. When you put words in, there's a demarcation. When you don't put words in, the nonverbal expression of the psyche just keeps going. So the word "expression," Maria, is the key when we're dealing with shadow – or anything else – but with the shadow particularly.

MARIA: Acceptance of the expression of –

LUCIA: Expression is absolute key.

KAY: I disagree. It's the experience that does it, not the expression.

LUCIA: Oh – oh, okay. All right.

MARIA: But, you have to express in order to experience.

KAY: It's experience of expression.

ALL: Yea-a-ah! [clapping and laughter]

MARIA: And there's something that's easier about accepting the experience of the expression of the shadow than it is to interact with it. And what we're saying about the nonverbal is important because with the verbal we may get caught.

LUCIA: Mm-hmm.

MARIA: Now I am reflecting back to my own sandplay process, to one of the last trays I created. And after all these years, there is a profound image from that tray, that I'm still integrating. I am sure both of you have had this kind of experience. Growing up Italian Catholic, the Virgin Mary was so prevalent. And I remember this particular tray where I had the Virgin Mary and Kali, face to face, with a little flower between them, a little tiny flower, that emerged out of that face-to-face connection between those two archetypal feminine, spiritual figures. Looking back I see the opposites in which one is the shadow and one is the Self.

KAY: They are of each other.

MARIA: It's a profound coming together, for me, of the shadow and the Self. It's my personal, familial, and cultural experience of the yin–yang.

LUCIA: Yes.

MARIA: The tension of those two figures is so deep. There is the tension of the opposites. It is so profound what reverberates in us when we create a sandtray, when all the levels of our psyche are engaged in and experience this expression. And then, it's a lifetime of integration.

KAY: Well, you've told about your shadow experience so I will tell you the image from my sandtray. I put a witch looking into the mirror. And to me, at the time, it didn't mean very much. That's the reason I'm so hipped on experience. Because, after that, my relationship with my sister – about which I went to Dora to do sandplay – got better. I didn't know why. I just thought it was something else until Dora and I went over my trays together, ten years later. And then I realized without her telling me, that the mirror was reflecting back to me the witchy part of myself. And that was so profound to me. I was experiencing my shadow. It had been working in me all that time.

MARIA: Yes. So you have that image and you'll never forget it.

KAY: Yes. And it helped me without my being conscious of it. It helped me without Dora's saying anything about it. If she had, I probably would have rejected it. I was very rejecting of the idea that our problem had anything to do with me.

MARIA: Except you went there to work on it.

KAY: That's true. My psyche made me go to work on it, but at a conscious level I wanted to find out that our problem was all her fault.

LUCIA: Well, since we're telling Dora stories, I am remembering one of the trays I created with Dora. I didn't think of it as shadow but I'm beginning to realize that maybe it was. I did a tray with Dora, and it was quite a pretty tray. There were cultivated fields and there was a big expanse of water, and there was a sailboat on the water. In talking to her about it, I said, "It's rudderless." And she said, "What's that?" And I said, "It doesn't have a way to go any place." And she said to me, "Ah, that is your dark." And I didn't have a clue what she meant about that but here I am, with my schedule book, scheduled up for the next two years, avoiding just being rudderless out in the ocean. Oh, that's hard.

KAY: Mine was hard, too.

MARIA: Except you both experienced something getting better, probably, in your making a relationship to the shadow.

KAY: Yes, but it's kind of hard to – to acknowledge. But I – I have. I do. But it took how many years?

LUCIA: I know. That's it, isn't it? The depth that we're talking about, for shadow material, is that you keep going into it, forever.

KAY: It isn't a done thing.

MARIA: Well, yeah, we keep working with the witch energy or the rudderless energy or the Kali energy. I realized that my identification was with the Virgin Mary and that was just pure innocence. But Kali has me facing the rage and destruction in myself and in the world. And making room for it.

KAY: Beautiful.

LUCIA: And it still is with you. The image is just as clear as the day you did it.

MARIA: Ah! I can see it.

KAY: I can see it.

LUCIA: I can see it, too. There, you see that's the guts to guts.

MARIA: So facing the shadow in sandplay has a profound impact on us and on our own individuation process.

LUCIA: Yeah, it takes a little bit of guts, doesn't it? So that old radio program, I talked about earlier, was true: The shadow knows. The shadow knows about our completion in some way. And we must know the shadow to be complete.

KAY: And the song "Me and My Shadow" is right too. The shadow is always with us.

Chapter 22

Shadow

Maria Ellen Chiaia

> The shadow usually presents a fundamental contrast to the conscious personality. This contrast is the prerequisite for the difference of potential from which psychic energy arises. Without it, the necessary tension would be lacking. Where considerable psychic energy is at work, we expect a corresponding tension and inner opposition. The opposites are necessarily of a characterological nature: the existence of a positive virtue implies victory over its opposite, the corresponding vice; without its counterpart, virtue would be pale, ineffective and unreal. The extreme opposition of the shadow to consciousness is mitigated by complementary and compensatory processes in the unconscious. The impact on consciousness finally produces the uniting symbols.
>
> (Jung, 1963, par. 707)

This process that Jung describes so beautifully is experienced through expression in the sand and later may be viewed in the sand pictures. This tension and inner opposition between conscious and unconscious and the resulting uniting symbols appear over and over again throughout a sandplay process.

As sandplay therapists we hold a space open, in deep relationship to ourselves and to the other, for this process to unfold. We look for the oppositions and the tensions from tray to tray. We also observe these oppositions within a tray. I pay attention to which figures are placed diagonally across from one another. For example, a group of fighting animals may be placed in the upper left corner and a Buddha and a Kuan-Yin may be placed in the lower right. In this scene there is a feeling of tension between aggressive instinctual energies and a quiet, compassionate spiritual energy. And from this opposition something new may arise which unites this energy for the sandplayer. In a future tray, a peasant woman living alone in the forest with bears and other wild animals appears. As a uniting symbol, she is a human being who lives and works in nature, in solitude, and has a relationship to animals. The person creating this sandplay may be experiencing a feminine spirituality connected to the earth and her creatures and the oppositions within have given way to this new experience.

Or this tension may be seen in two figures placed face to face or back to back. As stated in the shadow trialogue (Chapter 21), in my sandtray, when the Virgin faced Kali, I experienced this opposition and it upset my conscious experience of spirituality and the feminine. And out of that tension a red flower emerged. As a uniting symbol the red flower holds a growing, feeling aliveness which became part of my vegetative body. The simple, biological, organism that is "I" began to feel a range of emotions connected to my spirituality and my experience of the feminine that had not been available before.

I also note the order that figures go into a single tray. One figure placed in the tray and then another that is opposite the first figure may suggest that energies are in opposition and are trying to resolve. For example, fire is placed in the tray followed by water; and then a furnace followed by an igloo; then a stove followed by a refrigerator; then an ice pond followed by a fireplace. All of these go into the tray. In this example psychic energies are building as extreme opposites are being experienced in this expression. We must watch closely for what may arise from this, either in this tray or in the next. The sandplay and the therapeutic relationship are holding these opposing energies as a whole and accepting them. The uniting symbol will appear as the conscious is being impacted by the unconscious.

Jung describes this process so well when he compares what happens in the psyche to what happens in alchemy.

> But if his recognition of the shadow is as complete as he can make it, then conflict and disorientation ensue, an equally strong Yes and No which he can no longer keep apart by a rational decision . . . It requires a real solution and necessitates a third thing in which the opposites can unite. Here the logic of the intellect usually fails, for in a logical antithesis there is no third. The "solvent" can only be an irrational nature. In nature the resolution of opposites is always an energic process: she acts *symbolically* in the truest sense of the word, doing something that expresses both sides, just as a waterfall visibly mediates between above and below. The waterfall itself is then the incommensurable third. In an open and unresolved conflict dreams and fantasies occur which, like the waterfall, illustrate the tension and nature of the opposites, and thus prepare the synthesis.
>
> (1963, par. 705)

Jung recommends that we work with a process that bypasses our logical, rational mind in order for the third, the uniting symbol, to arise. He would ask his patients to create a series of images in order to reveal the contents of the unconscious. By dealing with these contents, he knew that the patient would come face to face with the "other," which he likened to the shadow. Over and over again, Jung witnessed how this process would enable the patient to gain insight into the complex nature of the personality through the images that emerged. And how through these images a third thing would be created and the opposites would be united.

In sandplay the sand, water and miniatures call to us, bypassing our rational minds. The creation that emerges expresses the tension and nature of the opposites, and also allows for a synthesis to occur. And it is not only expressed but also experienced by the sandplayer and the therapist. Sandplay engages our unconscious, creating a bridge to consciousness. In creating sandtrays we actively make a relationship between the ego and the Self, the persona and the shadow, the shadow and the Self. By engaging the known and the not known, the seen and the unseen, something new emerges which is the product of our imagination, coming from the deep unconscious. When the psyche has access to these energies from the unconscious, the shadow is engaged and both the unconscious and the conscious are impacted and transformed. And as stated in the trialogue, we become more three-dimensional and more filled-out as human beings the more we can live in relationship to those parts of ourselves that are less conscious or split off.

Chapter 23

Shadow

Kay Bradway

The "shadow" is a somewhat shadowy concept that seems to elude final definition or even stable description. Jung first defined his concept of shadow in a 1915 publication as the "negative side of the personality, the sum of all those unpleasant qualities we like to hide, together with the insufficiently developed functions and the contents of the personal unconscious" (Jung, 1953, par. 103, fn 5).

By 1959, Jung had expanded his concept of the shadow. He writes:

> It has been believed hitherto that the human shadow was the source of all evil. It can now be ascertained on closer investigation that the unconscious man, that is, his shadow, does not consist only of morally reprehensible tendencies but also displays a number of good qualities, such as normal instincts, appropriate reactions, realistic insights, creative impulses, etc.
>
> (Jung, 1959, par. 423)

Jung's expansion of the shadow to include the positive, thus recognizing the psychological universality of the opposites, makes theoretical sense. The feeling tone associated with the word "shadow," however, continues to conjure up the negative. Some writers have described the shadow in terms of its being opposite to another psychological concept: to ego, to Self, to persona. But few have referred to the opposite, or positive, side of the shadow itself. An exception is Lucia Chambers's contribution in the shadow trialogue in this volume (Chapter 21).

After looking at a smattering of quotations from Jungian writers in the 1980s and 1990s, I would like to focus on the sandplay process of Debbie as an example of how shadow problems are handled with the use of visual images as distinguished from verbal dialogue.

In the 1982 edition of Murray Stein's book, *Jungian Analysis*, there are only two references to the shadow by any of the twenty-two contributing Jungian analysts. One is by Edward Whitmont, who alludes to the shadow's individual as opposed to cultural values: "We express the ideals of our family group and cultural environment, even when we hate or rebel against them or consciously disregard them. Genuinely individual values are more often than not carried by the shadow" (Stein, 1982, p. 337).

When a new edition of Stein's book was published in 1995 with the replacement of some of the authors by other Jungian analysts, the number of references to shadow showed an increase from two to thirteen. Stein himself, in observing only the negative side of the shadow, writes: "Becoming conscious of psychic parts of oneself that have hitherto been projected is a sobering and often a painful experience particularly when it involves aspects of the shadow, that portion of the personality that is disowned because of its unsavory and shameful desires and feelings" (p. 40).

Ann Ulanov writes of confrontation and integration of the shadow: "In confronting the shadow ... we see now how important it is to recollect at the same time what belongs to the ego." And "Recollection ... must go on simultaneously with shadow confrontation and integration" (Stein, 1995a, p. 59).

Donald Sandner and John Beebe write of the "classic Jungian concept" of the shadow as referring to the "part of the unconscious psyche that is closest to the consciousness, even though it is not fully acceptable to it" (Stein, 1995a, p. 304).

Sandner's and Beebe's discussion of psychic functions including the shadow notes that the "Split off parts of the shadow ... have been truly unconscious until they gradually emerge in dreams, symptoms or affects within the transference, seeking a relation with the patient's ego" (Stein, 1995a, pp. 344–345).

In his book on integrity, Beebe tells us of the importance of the shadow: "Experience with patients in psychotherapy teaches us that in the effort to restore integrity, facing the shadow is essential" (1992, p. 17).

Andrew Samuels' book *Jung and the Post-Jungians* was published in 1985, between the two editions of Stein's book. Samuels includes shadow in a discussion of "discrete archetypes" and alludes only to Jung's negative description of the shadow. He writes: "[Shadow is] a word coined by Jung to sum up what each man fears and despises and cannot accept in himself" (p. 31). And later, in a section entitled "Ego and shadow," Samuels says, "Jung used the term *shadow* to signify and sum up what each man fears and despises in himself." He goes on to say, "While it is possible for the ego to become conscious of what is located in the shadow, this can never be a total consciousness" (Samuels, 1985, p. 65).

A seminar entitled "Shadow and Self" given by Joseph Henderson in 1982, and included in his book of the same title published in 1990, is the most comprehensive contribution regarding the shadow. Henderson develops the idea that the shadow is not the opposite of the ego but the opposite of the Self. He notes that Jung envisioned "a continuous dialogue between manifestations of the shadow and the Self." Henderson adds that in his practice "there are three levels that this dialogue can take place: the personal, the cultural and the archetypal" (p. 69). He further offers that the shadow may be the opposite of the persona: "If there is such an entity as an ego, a concept upon which we are now casting some doubt, the outer aspect of it is the persona, that is, how we present ourselves to the world. The opposite of that persona is our shadow" (p. 71). In his analysis of a dream, Henderson equates self-doubt with a shadow problem.

And now for Debbie's sandplay process, which illustrates in images the confrontation of some shadow issues.

Debbie came to me to do sandplay in order to prepare for death. At our first meeting, she described the events leading up to the diagnosis of lung cancer and how her physician told her she would die within two years. She showed no affect in telling me all this. As I began to follow her sandplay process, I realized that besides coping with the death sentence, or perhaps more properly as part of coping with it, she had several problems to confront and handle: her ambivalence about religion, her trouble in dealing with fear and anger, negative projections onto her sister, negative images of her parents, feeling inferior as a woman, conflicts about attachments and detachments. I think Debbie's series of fourteen sandtrays shows both the confrontation and finally a resolution of several of these problems, some of which had been issues for her for many years. The following observations are only a small portion of the full analysis of Debbie's process which appears in Bradway and McCoard (1997, pp. 201–212).

Debbie did not have a secure religious belief to help her in her preparation for death. She described herself as an agnostic. In her initial tray, however, she placed a Madonna, explaining to me when she added the Madonna as the final item, that she had not wanted to include it because she was suspicious of all Christian symbols, but something in her made her put it in anyway.

As she made her initial tray, and before she added the Madonna, she seemed to be denying all fear and anger about her death sentence. She used items connected with immortality and with spontaneous regeneration or healing. By the third tray, made immediately after making a benign, comforting tray, she was able to fully experience her fears and anger. She started the tray by putting in a figure that is often seen as a diabolic representation of death and she called it "frightening." After adding a black bat below it, she added five figures of Bodhidharmas, truncated human bodies without legs or eyelids, and called them "nightmarish." These figures may have reflected Debbie's fear of bodily deterioration, which in persons with cancer may be as great a fear as that of death. Debbie placed other frightening figures in the tray as well: a leering face, a ghoulish head, alligators. Near some mice she added a witch, a negative mother image which may have been associated with her personal mother and/or with me. I was sitting at the corner of the tray closest to where she placed the witch. Five aggressively armed soldiers added near the last may have stood for her anger. In the sandtray she could concretize both her fear and anger in the safety of the co-transference. She never talked directly at any point in the sandplay series about either of these emotions. Expressing and experiencing them in the sandplay process was enough.

In her fourth tray Debbie placed two wrestlers and commented on the fights she used to have with her sister. She could not remember what they fought about but she just remembered they were always fighting. I find that sisters, especially if they are the only siblings, often provide for shadow projection. After I fully recognized this in my own relationship with my older sister, I was more able to note it in my clients. In Debbie's case, the wrestling figures may have been preparing the ground for further confrontation and resolution. They reappeared in a tray toward the end of her process along with the reappearance of other images of fear. I recalled von Franz's interpreting the image of wrestlers in a dream of a dying patient as a wrestling with death. Debbie's earlier struggle with her personal shadow may have extended now to the larger struggle with death (an archetypal shadow?).

In the tray that immediately followed, Debbie concretized anger in the form of an active volcano that explodes fire, and then countered it in the form of an incense burner that securely contains fire. I saw this as an example of confrontation and then resolution.

Other shadow problems were worked on and resolved in a similar way. Several successive trays showed a working at a conscious/unconscious level on her differentiation between the genders and her envy of the masculine. Finally she made a scene that depicted a resolution of her long-held feeling of inferiority to males. It was in one of her later trays that she made a large body of water in the center of the tray with a small island emerging from the water. The sun shines on the island on which are two babies, one wrapped in blue and the other in pink, a boy and a girl. It is as if the sun, representing consciousness, has come forth from the waters of the unconscious and, with this rise in consciousness, Debbie comes to experience the masculine and feminine as equals.

Her conflict about "attachment/detachment" was worked out both through the co-transference and in her trays. At one point, when I was about to take a vacation, she began the hour by saying that she wanted to stop for a while, which clearly was making it possible for her to dismiss me before I dismissed her, in this way denying the attachment. She claimed she hadn't remembered that I was going on my vacation. It was in doing this tray that she portrayed recognizable breasts, despite her voiced wish not to have them look like breasts; breasts could reflect dependency and attachment (described in more detail in the Mother trialogue in this volume).

The working out of negative relationships with her parents was also shown in the trays. Finally she was able to make a tray in which both mother and father figures were seen in a protecting way. She recalled her mother's care of her when she had a kidney operation and added, "You need a mother when you feel sick."

In her final tray, done shortly before her death, Debbie included the same Madonna she had used reluctantly in her initial tray, but this time she honored it by placing it on a crescent moon which rests on the earth. She also included her frequently used beaded snake that she had identified as her "intimate being," but in this tray she coiled the snake in a counterclockwise coil in contrast to her previously always coiling this snake in a clockwise direction. The clockwise direction is traditionally recognized as traveling in the direction of consciousness whereas the counterclockwise direction is recognized as traveling in the direction of the unconscious. I felt that Debbie sensed or was experiencing at this point that at death there is an inversion, an inversion of the known and the unknown. At death the known, the ego identity, the "I," becomes the unknown; the personal ego-snake goes down and disappears into the unconscious. And the other, the up there, the unknowable, becomes, at death, the known.

This tray was done at Debbie's final visit to my office. I saw her a few times in her home before she died. Debbie died at home. Her son described her death as "peaceful, with little need of pain killers until the very last."

Chapter 24

Shadow

Lucia Chambers

I have a little shadow that goes in and out with me,
And what can be the use of him is more than I can see.

R.L. Stevenson, from "My Shadow"

Living with others, of animal or human species, requires the establishment of a set of standards and rules, a structure that provides a sense of security from the forces that pose a threat to the existence of all members of the group. Some of these forces are an objective reality such as provided by life itself with its seeming randomness of happenings, and by nature with her uncontrollable, fearsome powers. Other forces are of a subjective nature. Individually or collectively, sometimes a judgment is made that a certain person, a group of people, a behavior, or another set of standards is a menace to the preexisting structure. These threatening forces, seen as "other," often are seen as evil. There can be cohesiveness in a group when people agree that a particular group or ideology is evil. In these group psyche situations, there evolves the undifferentiated experience of a common enemy. In this huddle, we believe that we are safe from "them." But there is terrible danger! As the group huddles together, it works to strengthen the barriers against the perceived threat. It might begin to try to eliminate the evil or the "other." Moving together, the collective begins to be destructive. Believing itself to be "good," it has assumed the very energies that were judged as "bad" in the "other." Peck says, "Strangely enough, evil people are often destructive because they are trying to destroy evil. The problem is that they misplace the locus of evil. Instead of destroying others, they should be destroying the sickness within themselves" (1983, p. 74).

Jung clarifies, "We must beware of thinking of good and evil as absolute opposites" (Abrams and Zeig, 1991, p. 74). He says:

First and foremost, the individual has need of Self knowledge, that is, the utmost possible knowledge of his own wholeness. He must know relentlessly how much good he can do, and what crimes he is capable of, and must beware of regarding the one as real and the other as an illusion. Both are elements within his nature.

(Abrams and Zeig, 1991, p. 172)

The Self, by definition, is our unique totality. But there are some parts of ourselves that threaten the development of our identity as it is shaped by our childhood experiences. Our understanding of what is good is internalized by praise, pleasure and temperament; what is bad through punishment, shame and guilt. In our need to belong to the group and to find safety there, we make similar judgments about those good and bad aspects when we find them within ourselves. We deny them, reject them and thrust them into the dark of our unconscious. And sometimes, in a desperate effort to disown them, we project them onto others.

Compelled by an enormous amount of defensive energy, we talk and ruminate endlessly on the shocking nature of other people, institutions or ideologies. We might be compelled to act out our fear in some destructive way. Hesse says in his great book *Demian* that if you hate a person, you hate something in him that is a part of yourself. What isn't part of ourselves doesn't disturb us (1976). An interesting facet of this phenomenon is that the rejected parts of ourselves might be the more positive aspects of our personality. The projection onto the "other" might be that of wisdom or gentleness or beauty or spirituality. We still are separating out a part of our Self, rejecting it and relegating it to the unknown.

A radio program from the 1940s began each episode with the chilling words "What evil lurks in the hearts of men? The Shadow knows!" Our shadow does "know." It holds all of our unlived potential. The path of individuation, or self-realization, is the arduous and painful path of reclaiming the parts of ourselves that the ego has repressed as unacceptable, the parts that do not fit the ego-ideal. Jung said that truthfully the shadow is 90 percent pure gold (Abrams and Zeig, 1991). Paradoxically, the ego becomes what is wrong and the shadow becomes what is right and what can provide the healing. This might be a response to Robert Louis Stevenson's poem "My Shadow" (1944). Mining for the gold then becomes a struggle: a struggle that we experience as suffering. We might have physical ailments ranging from the more mild headaches and body pain to diseases which threaten life itself. Or we might have psychological "illness" ranging from irritability and emotional outbursts to debilitating depression. These symptoms tell us, if we are willing to listen, that the Self is attempting to direct our consciousness to an awareness of a rejected side of the personality. These neglected aspects must be accepted despite the resistance of the ego in order to establish a new order, a transformed identity. In the sand, this struggle is recognized as a necessary part of the process of healing and held without being pulled into the judgmental shadow energy.

Suffering is acknowledged as containing an "element of the divine" (Corbett, 1996, p. 51). It is religious. The meaning of the word "religion" is *re*, meaning again, and *ligature*, meaning bind or bridge. This religious aspect of the psyche can be welcomed by the sandplay therapist who knows that the darkest moment always comes before the dawning of new light. The Self is there bringing together again the very parts of our soul that we have reviled. In this moment, the sandplay therapist can contribute, in a minute way, to the lessening of the moral darkness of the world.

> This thing of darkness I
> Acknowledge mine.
> > William Shakespeare,
> > *The Tempest*, Act V Scene 1

Part VII

Chaos

Chapter 25

Chaos trialogue

LUCIA: How to talk about Chaos? I have to go right back to Jung to help me sort out this kind of thing. He is such a gift to me! The first thing I think of is opposites, so there is dark and light. So, if I'm talking about the dark then there must be light. There must be. And if I'm talking about chaos, there must be order. So that's very positive, don't you think? It doesn't scare you, like CHAOS! Okay, where's the light?

MARIA: Well, I think about darkness as being an absence of light, and in order to have darkness, you have to have light.

KAY: In order to have light, you have to have darkness.

LUCIA: But that's necessary, isn't it?

MARIA: Right. Exactly. I think about the beginning of the Bible in which there was darkness and then there was light. So it is creation.

LUCIA: In Buddhist theory, too, it's chaos first. Out of the chaos comes –

MARIA: The order.

KAY: Well, you can't see the stars until it's dark. This was so exciting when I first realized this. No night, no stars. No dark, no light.

LUCIA: That's right. It has to get to be dark. And then the stars are their own kind of light, aren't they?

KAY: Light and darkness complement each other. That is the theory of opposites. And if you go so far in one direction, you get –

LUCIA: Enantiodromia. Love that word.

KAY: Wonderful! Then – you get the other. And if you only have the light all the time, then it can't be.

LUCIA: It's not possible, is it?

KAY: No. Or in the darkness all the time. When you're very depressed, you know that there will be light.

LUCIA: That's all right, Kay, but how about when you're very happy and feeling very light? Then what comes next? I'm thinking of the stars. Here in the city, where there's so much light, you can't see the stars.

KAY: Right.

LUCIA: So you have to seek out the dark. You have to go to a place that is very, very dark before you can see those stars.

KAY: And that's the whole thing.

LUCIA: I'm wondering if this isn't a metaphor. You have to go into the darkness, and the further into the dark you go, the more brilliant becomes the light – when you find it.

MARIA: Jung talks about the doctrine of the *lumen naturae*, which states that nature contains a luminosity. In the depths and the darkness of the unconscious are sparks of light, in the dark are soul sparks. The fishes' eyes, *scintillae*, are depicted as eyes in the stars, in the earth, in the water, or in nature. Here is the light in the darkness.

LUCIA: Fish eyes! Why does he call it fish eyes?

MARIA: *Lumen naturae* is light in nature and that light is depicted as eyes. His idea comes from different alchemical texts. Many references are made to eyes and one of the texts speaks of *oculi piscium*, fishes' eyes. Swimming around in the darkness of the unconscious, there's the light of consciousness in the eyes of the fish. The sun is the light of consciousness and the *lumen naturae* is light in nature in the unconscious.

LUCIA: If we think about the individuation process, where would we put darkness and chaos in that? We see chaos in the sand all the time. It frequently appears in the trays of abused children.

KAY: Well, I get suspicious if I get too many trays and there is no chaos in them. I really kind of wonder.

MARIA: When they are all neat and pretty.

KAY: Yeah.

LUCIA: So what are you saying?

KAY: I feel that for growth, for individuation, or if someone comes because they are in pain, and there is no chaos in the trays then I wonder.

MARIA: So there's something about being willing to go into the darkness.

KAY: Needing to.

MARIA: But if one is just ambitious and goal-oriented around the sandplay, there's not going to be a need to go there.

LUCIA: I *never* want to go there! I don't care if I'm going to be enlightened or not!

KAY: You can't help yourself. A person comes to therapy because they're in pain. And the psyche knows this. The psyche knows that you're paying good money for it and the psyche goes that way. It'll get you into the chaos.

LUCIA: So you have to have a need.

MARIA: For what?

KAY: To develop. To get over your pain.

MARIA: When I started with Jungian analysis, I was wanting something that Jung could articulate beyond any possibility that I could get at. Once I got into it, I went right down into the pain. And it was like, "Oh my God, if I knew it was going to be like this, I never would have gone."

KAY: Why did I get into this?

LUCIA: I'm thinking of the diagram Estelle Weinrib uses to describe the sandplay process. We leave the conscious level and we descend. And it's not so bad at first. The animals come in and there are plants and rocks. That's not so bad. And then, if you keep on, you will descend into a place where there is a rearrangement of all the elements as they were existing up to this point in time, and that means a letting go. And you can't let go and know that something else is coming. So you have to let go into nothingness. You let go into chaos. The ego does. And then there is this time – Jung called it "dark night of the soul" – when there is nothing there. The old is gone and the new is not there yet.

MARIA: And I think that's where the relationship to the therapist comes in. Because the therapist has been through this and holds the possibility that something will emerge.

KAY: And you have to trust that this relationship will hold you until you can let go. It's like swimming and you're hanging onto a rope and you let go of the rope. Where did it go? The ocean comes in. You have to trust that there is someone there.

LUCIA: And if you are going into it, you can't believe it's going to be okay.

KAY: Or it won't work. I've tried it.

ALL: [laughter]

LUCIA: And so the sandplay therapist holds the darkness.

KAY: Holds the darkness – *and* the lightness.

MARIA: Or holds the possibility that something will come of the darkness and the chaos.

LUCIA: Yes.

MARIA: It's a tricky thing because my sense of it is clinging to the hope but also being in the darkness with the sandplayer.

LUCIA: The therapist can't run away either.

MARIA: The therapist can't move too much into the hope either.

LUCIA: No. You have to stay right there at that edge.

KAY: Yes, but the psyche knows.

MARIA: It knows. But sometimes when I'm holding the hope, I'm not sure that the sandplayer can do it. I sometimes work with people who are suicidal. They might ask, "Are you holding the hope for me?" And I say, "Yes." But at times there is so much despair that I wonder if they will come out of it. Although I know from experience that people do. So, it's this strange place of being with the hope but at the same time knowing that some people don't make it.

LUCIA: Of course we hold the hope that they will feel better and be enlightened and all that. But more importantly, we hold the faith that whatever happens is the right thing. Jung found that in the psychosis, in the psychotic hallucinations, is the truth, living in concealed form.

MARIA: Right.

LUCIA: So maybe even psychosis is the right thing.

KAY: Oh, yes. Psychosis is not always to be avoided.

MARIA: Psychosis is not to be avoided any more than suicidal ideation.

LUCIA: So what is the right thing? What do you hope for?

MARIA: It's like that glimmer of light – keeping that glimmer of light alive, that there is a light there – what it is – where it's going.

LUCIA: The form that it's going to take.

KAY: Well, I hope that there is a change. But when a person makes the same tray over and over and over again, it's kind of hard to hold the experience in your mind that they will change.

LUCIA: So, it's hope for change.

KAY: It's knowledge. It's belief. It isn't that I believe it; I know it. I *know* there will be a change.

LUCIA: So, it's waiting for the change, then. What are we doing when we are sitting with the dark and we are looking at these horrendous trays and the client is in terrible pain?

KAY: Seeing the tray gives me the experience and therefore I can really hold the faith or hope or whatever.

MARIA: That's right. Then you can hold onto something. There's something in the psyche that is moving. In the sandplay, you look in the tray and there is total chaos, for example just some teacups are upright and everything else is dumped all over. But in one corner, you see something hopeful.

KAY: And we know they're coping with it – that this tray is coping.

LUCIA: The tray is?

KAY: That those images are the client's way – at that moment – to cope with what they are feeling.

LUCIA: That's right! You got it.

KAY: And so – if the coping goes on, then that's all we can do. I always remember Joe Henderson's "Trust the process." That has helped me many times. Of course, it is critical that we be sufficiently trained and experienced so that we know when we must protect sandplayers from physically harming themselves or others.

MARIA: But even in the chaos you'll see something.

KAY: You'll see something what?

MARIA: Of the – what you were saying – in the darkness is the path. Sometimes, you'll see something of the path.

KAY: Even if there isn't, though. Supposing there isn't?

LUCIA: But isn't there always?

KAY: Well, I wouldn't need to see that there was anything.

MARIA: You don't *need* to see.

KAY: No.

MARIA: At that point you don't need to see. You're right.

KAY: No.

LUCIA: You just know that something is happening.

MARIA: You're right. You're right.

KAY: In fact, I think if I do see something, that's kind of a false –

LUCIA: That's not the point?

KAY: That's right. It's not the point. It's just the chaos. It's just there. As I said, it's their way of coping. I don't have to see anything happening.

LUCIA: So, you have absolute faith in the process that is happening in the sand.

KAY: At that moment. The thing that is hardest to put up with is when there is no change. So sometimes there is no chaos. But if there were no chaos, I would accept it too. You can't do anything but accept it.

LUCIA: Yes you can. They are given pills all the time.

ALL: [laughter]

KAY: True.

LUCIA: I'm thinking of how the mental health profession is avoiding the dark and the chaos by medicating.

KAY: Exactly. Exactly.

LUCIA: Across the board, medicating out that experience. And what happens? Something like Columbine happens. Somehow that darkness is going to demand to be acknowledged. And if we don't acknowledge it, recognize it, and be there – with faith in the change, then it will be like anything repressed, it'll simply get bigger and come out in another place.

KAY: It will explode.

LUCIA: I really do believe that Columbine and September 11 were symptoms of what we are doing now, which is not honoring the dark and the chaos as the place that is necessary before the creation begins.

MARIA: Just the image – of this ash, black ash all over, and people breathing it – and in that ash there are human bodies. Everything that we kept sanitized was not sanitized. It had to be faced –

LUCIA: You have to acknowledge that it's there.

MARIA: Exactly.

LUCIA: And be willing to stand in relationship to it. To accept that it is there – and not just push it under the rug.

KAY: And, as you say, we give pills to make it disappear. Everyone wants it nice.

LUCIA: That's right. Everything has to be nice.

KAY: Sanitized.

LUCIA: And the nicer it gets, the blacker the black – and the more chaotic the chaos.

MARIA: There is an alchemical drawing that shows a dog and a wolf fighting. This image has tremendous chaotic energy.

LUCIA: Absolutely.

MARIA: The yin–yang, it has the light in the dark and the dark in the light. It's all there.

LUCIA: That's right. Life *must* contain the dark as well as the light.

MARIA: If it's the whole, then it contains everything.

KAY: The Self is wholeness, but it contains those two opposites in a way that is very difficult for the human ego to contain.

MARIA: Because, in any kind of sandplay process, we are providing a free and protected space for the opposites of both darkness and light, chaos and order.

LUCIA: I wonder if our beautiful logical minds are at work. Culturally the dark is bad and so needs to be avoided.

KAY: Okay. And so?

LUCIA: In the "beginning," dark was –

KAY: It.

LUCIA: That's right. So, again, in the sand, we step out of the brain that wants to organize and prioritize things; and we step back into the place where there is *everything* and the dark is just as important as the light in the process of creation. I think that is something that really needs to be looked at. We've lost the valuing of the dark.

MARIA: In sandplay, we provide a space where the darkness and the chaos are valued; it is of tremendous value in the process.

LUCIA: It is so important to put in here, that the sandplay therapist has to have had the experience of the dark. We have to know what it is like to be lost in the chaos and where everything is awful, and then to have to come up out of it. Then we will be able to acknowledge the value of the ugly, dark trays. We have to *know* that the dark is an essential part of the new thing that is going to come. It's almost like a reverence.

KAY: Respect.

LUCIA: Respecting the dark.

Chapter 26

Chaos

Maria Ellen Chiaia

> Man's inner life is the "secret place" . . . the spark of the light in nature . . .
> Those labouring in the darkness must try to accomplish an opus that will
> cause the "fishes' eyes" to shine in the depths of the sea, or to catch the
> "refracted rays of the divine majesty" even though this produces a light
> which the darkness, as usual, does not comprehend . . . For the darkness
> has its own peculiar intellect and its own logic, which should be taken
> seriously. Only the "light which the darkness comprehendeth not" can
> illuminate the darkness. Everything that the darkness thinks, grasps, and
> comprehends by itself is dark; therefore it is illuminated only by what, to it,
> is unexpected, unwanted, and incomprehensible. The psychotherapeutic
> method of active imagination offers excellent examples of this.
>
> (Jung, 1963, pars 344–345)

In sandplay the imagination of the sandplayer unfolds in the creation of a
sandtray. We as sandplay therapists value the chaos and darkness as the
unexpected, unwanted and incomprehensible, and from this the "fishes' eyes"
may shine and begin to illuminate the path. Jung is telling us that what we do
not know, understand, or want holds the possibility of illumination. The
expression in a sandtray of what we do not know, understand or want begins
to shine like the "fishes' eyes" or the sparks of light in nature – the *lumen
naturae*. Herein is where we find the hope and the meaning. In the creation of
a sandtray, the expression and experience of the images of the unconscious
emerge, thereby containing and creating the possibility of illumination. Not
by the light of rationality or reason, but by "illumination of a degree and
kind that are equal to the darkness but are the exact opposite of 'enlightenment'"(Jung, 1963, par. 343).

Enlightenment, as Jung is using it here, means the light of reason. An
illumination that may be equal to the darkness must spring from suffering,
pain or an insoluble dilemma or conflict, when the latent autonomy of the
unconscious becomes active. Then doing sandplay becomes a need and the
sandplay therapist provides the container and the free and protected space so
the sandplayer can let go and let the unconscious lead. The trays can be

frightening, overwhelming, terrifying; and all this is accepted and held by the therapist who knows that something is being experienced in the darkness and chaos and that something is also emerging in the experience of darkness and chaos.

Trays depicting dismemberment appear during this time. One must dismember to remember: one must de-structure to restructure. The Tower card in the Crowley Tarot deck exemplifies this archetype: a building is on fire and disintegrating; a dove holding a branch emerges from the flames. When chaos and darkness have consumed us, then the destruction of our world as we know it, whether by floodwaters or fire, must occur so that new possibilities or new ways of experiencing this chaos and darkness may rise up from the unknown. Jung states that "the motif of dismemberment . . . is well known in alchemy. The atoms are or become 'white sparks' shining in the *terra foetida* (the fetid earth). They are also called the 'fishes' eyes' " (Jung, 1963, par. 64). This experience is identical with the stage of the *nigredo* in alchemy, the stage of darkness or chaos. So again we see that in the darkness there is light or illumination, the meaning from the unknowing that may emerge from the unconscious.

Rage and anger are part of this realm of chaos and darkness. Both rage and anger are destructive forces that seek to tear up, break apart, kill off and dismember. This is the realm of Kali, the Hindu goddess of creation and destruction. She is fiery red and stands on corpses and drinks blood; sometimes in images of Kali all we see are her eyes, as symbols of consciousness in darkness. There is illumination that comes from fiery rage and anger.

A woman, Laura, with whom I worked for many years entered into hatred and anger and destructive rage. The following epigram is from an alchemical text, *Atalanta Fugiens*.

> The wolf comes from the sunrise, but from where
> It sets there comes the dog, both wild with rage.
> Now each one bites the other, bites in fury,
> Their muzzles gaping in a rabid snarl.
> These are the twin stones, freely given you
> In all things and at all times; grasp them well.
>
> Maeir, 1989

This is the field Laura and I entered together.

Laura suffered extreme abuse. As these cases go, the abuse and rage entered into our relationship and the sandplay. In this chaotic sandtray (Figure 26.1), the rage and anger are experienced in the following figures: the volcano in the center of the tray, the large shark, the snakes, Kali, the aggressive dinosaurs, devils and monsters. The figures were thrown in, with some figures threatening others.

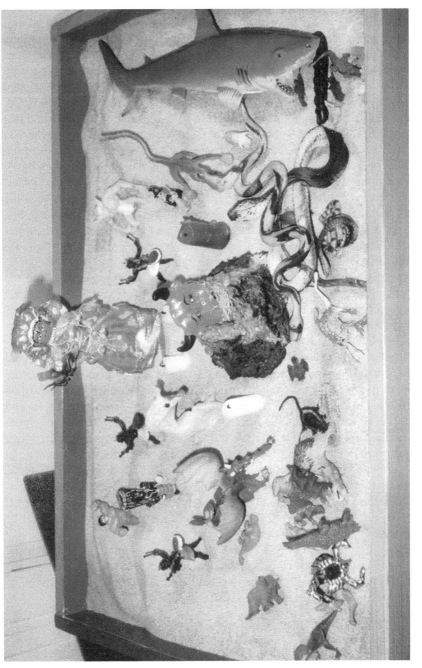

Figure 26.1 A tray by Laura

For many months the destructive rage entered in, trying to destroy one of the only safe places we had once created together. She threatened to quit therapy, yelled and broke things. I worked hard, working with containing my own destructive impulses and my desire to retaliate, appropriate co-transference responses. All the time I was allowing myself to meet this energy and contain it with Laura. When she could get into the sand, she created many chaotic and dark trays, leaving the trays destroyed and dismembered. There was great value in these sandplays as Laura's anger had protected her, helped her survive and kept her inner spirit alive and safe. Her anger was appropriate given what she experienced and in these trays she was connecting with archetypal energies of destruction and letting them move through her.

This all began to be worked through in Laura, and the light of the "fishes' eyes" became more and more brilliant. The *lumen naturae* began to shine and Laura became alive and connected to what was moving through her. She had needed to experience with me the abused and abusing self and the inner chaos in the sandplay. And the chaos led to a destructuring that allowed a transformation and something new to emerge.

About six months later, she did a sandtray. In this tray she honored the anger and rage in the large shark and in the figure of Kali, and yet we feel that healing and love have emerged in the figure of Kuan Yin, Chinese goddess of compassion, and the Virgin Mother and Child. We see the light of consciousness in the darkness by the candles illuminating her struggle for integration.

One Jungian analyst, Donald Kalsched (1996), speaks of these archetypal forces of darkness and chaos as demons that both protect and persecute those of us who have experienced trauma. He states that these forces must be confronted and humanized, in and through the relationship of therapist and client, as this was missing in the client's early relationships with caregivers. Certainly humanizing must occur so that the client does not identify with these forces and become negatively inflated. However, these are archetypal forces of darkness and chaos and they are not of us but exist in the universe. What we must do is to not become identified with them. They must be experienced in the sandplay and in dreams, and in the relationship to the therapist; but they must be allowed to move through us. They are forces that cannot be humanized as they exist in their own right.

These forces have a consciousness that must be illuminated through the light of the unconscious by being experienced in dreams and sandplay. Chaos and darkness have a light, a meaning, and a dark radiance that will shine if we create a space for their expression and experience.

Chapter 27

Chaos

Kay Bradway

Sandplay provides for the wordless expression and sharing of experiences of chaos and darkness that seem to defy full verbal description. The sharing of these experiences is a phase that people in depth therapy at one time or another encounter – *must* encounter. As a preliminary step sandplayers may need to create a tray that contains lightness, hope, even a symbol of the Self, before they can face the chaos or darkness. I have also found this in verbal analysis, but it is more apparent to me when I am using sandplay. On the other hand, sometimes after a tray showing chaos or darkness, sandplayers need to quickly make another tray that brings them back up to a place of light. They can't leave the hour safely, perhaps, without providing themselves with this ability, knowledge, experience, of coming back.

The chaos or darkness may be shown in many different ways, all pointing to the same depth of feelings of hopelessness, being destroyed, the end. For some it may be fighting and destroying, for some all dark objects, for some a multiplicity of objects – sometimes it seems as if a client is bent on taking all the items off your shelves and putting or throwing them into the tray. Sometimes it's pouring in volumes of water – if this hasn't been done previously. Therapists recognize the darkness by their own feelings of the hopelessness that is happening in the tray. There is often a numinous feeling about the tray at this moment, just as when a so-called Self tray appears. The Self tray is an experience of wholeness. A chaos/darkness tray may be an experience of emptiness even if it is full of items. It is different for each sandplayer. There is no standardized description or formula. I'd like to give three examples of what I have observed.

A young woman who knew that she would have only five sessions to do sandplay was able to include her drop into the level of chaos/darkness by the third tray. One of the central focuses was the fighting between two large male gorillas. She said that they represented her anger. She also included a death figure. She put in more hopeful figures both before and after these placements, but there was clearly an atmosphere of having reached a dark area. The following tray was a coming up, and by her final tray she could reach her goal of connecting with the spiritual, which was through connecting with her child with whom she had been having intense difficulty. I felt there was a message here familiar to students of alchemy: the treasure lies in the *nigredo*.

Another example is that of a woman who had come following a diagnosis of lung cancer, with the physician's telling her that she had two years to live. In making the appointment she told me this in a flat tone with no sign of emotion. In our initial "get acquainted" visit, she was quite matter-of-fact and again showed no emotion. This was a woman who had just learned she had only two years to live. I shuddered a bit for her. Her first tray likewise did not reflect any of what I would have thought she must be feeling at some level. The second tray carried on some of the themes of the first tray, but again no darkness, no chaos. After she completed this tray, I found myself asking her if she would like to make another tray during this session. At that moment it seemed essential that I suggest this to her. And now it came out: the fear, the anger, the rage. I don't think she could have done this tray at this point unless she had done the previous tray, with its "niceness." This was the beginning of a meaningful process in which she dealt with her angry feelings, including those toward her father and toward her ex-husband. She was afraid of making new attachments, which, of course, included making an attachment to me.

A nine-year-old girl who was referred with a diagnosis of dyslexia took to the tray happily. She didn't want to talk, and didn't talk until much later in our time together. The tray in which I felt the chaos most distinctly did not appear until well into the series. She had previously had us do some shooting at each other with toy machine guns. And then she made a scene in which she used a large number of the miniatures from the shelves. They were not exactly placed "hit or miss," but they presented a scene that was far different from her previous ones. I experienced it as one of chaos. Her following scene was organized. Later, however, she returned to making a "negative" scene in which she portrayed a mother bawling out her daughter. She then put a cannon at the bottom aimed to shoot at this mother. This youngster's approach to chaos was not as definitive as in the two previous examples. She touched it several times and came back. This often happens. Usually it can't all be done in one session. One has to go there several times and come back. Sandplay therapists, because of their past experience, are able to stay there and be moved, even sometimes slightly frightened, but know at some deep place that this is necessary for this particular person at this particular time or it wouldn't be happening.

It's necessary to remember that therapists not only give the sandplayers freedom to do what they want to in the tray, but they are also responsible for protecting sandplayers from physically harming themselves or others. Therapists must know when they should seek help or consultation. The verbal therapy that is adjunctive to sandplay often provides a place to explore the advisability of seeking help.

Chapter 28

Chaos

Lucia Chambers

> Creation is as much destruction as construction.
>
> (Jung, 1969b, par. 245)

It is chaos! This is an exclamation that we use when no descriptive words or precise metaphor can convey the energy that is contained in a specific event. What we are seeing or what we are hearing has no order that is available to our intellectual understanding. Such understanding is the result of events or objects being organized singly or in clusters, and linked to some event or cluster by the reflecting consciousness of an individual. Then we have order and meaning. So we strive to find meaning in all things: in the seemingly random happenings of primal life. Lévi-Strauss writes:

> Scientists do tolerate uncertainty and frustration, because they must. The one thing they do not tolerate is disorder. The whole aim of theoretical science is to carry to the highest possible and conscious degree the perceptual reduction of chaos.
>
> (in Hillman, 1972, p. 99)

The extreme linear thinking of the Western world is driven by this fear of lack of understanding, of lack of order, of lack of meaning. With no understanding or order, there is no possibility to impose control on our world. We are prey to the intemperate passions of an angry God, or the random happenings of a haphazard life force, and we ourselves become incidental.

Chaos is portrayed in myth by the uncontrolled forces of nature, such as floods, fog, fire, hurricanes, raging ocean waters, or the "yawning abyss." These very same images are also used to represent the presence of God or a creative force. God speaks to Moses from a burning bush, and Noah has the task of creating a better humankind when the flood waters have cleansed the world of the old. Dorothy, in *The Wizard of Oz*, is carried to a new dimension by a tornado (Baum, 1900/1956).

In alchemy, chaos is the *prima materia* or the *massa confusa*, which a secret process could transform into gold. Chaos is the formless dark, original state where all connections are dissolved. There is no order. Nevertheless, all ingredients are still present in the one mass. This original mass is equivalent to the circle waiting for the attempt of the alchemist to distill out the gold, thus squaring the circle. This is the paradox of chaos. It is formless and carries form. It is death and carries life. It is destruction and carries construction. It is wounding and carries healing. Jung quotes Hölderlin: "Danger itself fosters the rescuing power" (1933, p. 220).

James Hillman tells us that "by refusing chaos . . . eros may also be lost" (1972, p. 99). Eros is an interior phenomenon which is, in itself, an absolute identification with the expressions of the soul, in other words, creativity. "Chaos and creativity are inseparable" (p. 99). As the lotus rising from the mud represents the emergence of light from the primordial slime and the phoenix rises regenerated from the ashes of its fire, so too the human psyche must suffer the pain and terror of destruction in order to rise transformed to a higher level of development.

Construction and destruction cannot be separated. Every creative act holds a death. "Soul-making entails soul-destroying" (Hillman, 1972, p. 37). This is an endless cycle which is encoded in the very essence of the living cosmos to insure its evolution. A theory was developed about this non-linear pattern in nature of certain behavior. Scientists called it "chaos theory." It was presented to the general public in a riveting science fiction thriller called *Jurassic Park*. In it, one of the characters is trying to explain to another his apprehension about the carefully contained prehistoric world they have created. He says, "Linearity is an artificial way of viewing the world . . . Life is actually a series of encounters in which one event may change those that follow in a wholly unpredictable, even devastating way. That's a deep truth about the structure of our universe. But for some reason we insist on behaving as if it were not true" (Crichton, 1990, p. 171). Earlier in the book he explains, "in any sort of complex system where there is confusion and unpredictability, we can find an underlying order" (p. 75). Even in chaos, where there seems to be overwhelming disorder, there is still a simple underlying principle. In the world of Jungian theory, this principle is the individuation process. This is a dynamic, living force, driven by the Self in its powerful desire to be actualized. When the individual or the collective has settled into repetitive, stultifying patterns, the Self may exhibit a ruthless energy that will overturn the status quo. The result may be experienced as chaos. The pain and fear can be great. We may try desperately to go back, to regain the lost sense of familiarity of the old order. But we cannot go back. The encoded principle of evolution will ever thrust us toward our own realization. There is an old Egyptian saying, "Willing or unwilling, the fates lead us to our destiny."

In the sandplay room, we may cringe when a tray is filled with many figures in haphazard positions, or a hand is swept across the sand picture scattering all the figures, or the miniatures are violently shoved under the sand. The therapist and the sandplayer are both in chaos. As therapists it is our task to remain present there, with courage and faith, and wait for the new order to emerge from the chaos.

> . . . each chaos mothers itself into form.
>
> Berry, 1990, p. 90

Part VIII

Numinous

Chapter 29

Numinous trialogue

MARIA: The numinous seems to be a very central part of sandplay therapy – making space for the numinous to occur. When I did my own sandplay process, what seemed to be an essential part of the experience was the opening to, connecting with, the numinous within myself and with my sandplay therapist. The whole experience of doing sand is a numinous experience, and this seems to have something to do with connecting with the silence, with the therapist and with the sand images. All of this comes as a powerful experience of one's own psyche, an experience which is different from thinking, talking or knowing something about the psyche. It's the experience of it – of the psyche.

LUCIA: I like what you said – the experience of connection.

MARIA: Connection between yourself – inner and outer.

LUCIA: The whole deal: life, the human species, archetypes of life – in all of its aspects. The marvelous thing is that with this connection, everything is okay, even with the shadowy dark. It is like when a mother comforts a child after the child has been hurt. She says, "It's going to be okay. It's fine. It's okay. It's okay." It's that feeling – for me.

MARIA: It's a feeling of the numinous or connection to the numinous. But the numinous is also about meaning, meaning in its deepest sense. My inner world is connected to my outer – and is resonant with meaning and connection.

KAY: We always want to find that we make sense – to ourselves. But that's at an intellectual level. This experience of the numinous is the same sort of thing, only not at a thinking level.

MARIA: Right.

KAY: But we make sense. Or the world makes sense. We talk about the word "mystery," but somehow when you get to that level, as you say, everything's all right.

MARIA: On the numinous level, we're connected up.

KAY: Yeah. We're just part of a – of a whole system. And we don't have to prove ourselves. We're all right just as we are.

MARIA: We're connected up to everything else and –

KAY: Really part of something.

MARIA: It connects.

LUCIA: It feels like it goes beyond the individual. Sometimes there are clients that I don't think I click very well with verbally. They don't seem to be doing too much, but when they do sand, there is a connection that's profound. Beyond the personal – beyond the little individual things that are difficult – there's still that connection. When someone does the sand, I am ready for the numinous to come.

KAY: You open a space for it.

LUCIA: I do. I do.

MARIA: So you open a space to meet and be met –

LUCIA: *Beyond* whatever else is going on between us.

KAY: In a way, *you* don't do it; your psyche does it. It isn't your ego that's doing it. It's your psyche, your unconscious, your Self. You don't have to *do* anything. Your system is doing it.

LUCIA: That's it.

MARIA: And that's why it's essential that we all have the experience of doing a sandplay process because you have to experience it in order to know it, have it happen, or open a space for it to happen.

KAY: That's it.

LUCIA: I have had – I'm sure you have too – a kind of extraordinary experience. My sand room is separate, a space in the back of the talking room. And when you go into this space, it's like stepping over the threshold. In the talking room, there's – sometimes there's a little disconnect, a little discord, a jangly feeling. But then, when we walk into the sand room, the jangly feeling just drops away.

MARIA: There's something about the numinosity of being in the room with the figures, for yourself, that sort of holds you in a space with the person.

LUCIA: And they know it too. There is a – I think it's maybe that the intention and the experiences that have happened in that room still linger there. And is it in my psyche or is it in the air, in the room or is it in the carpet, or what is it?

MARIA: Maybe the experiences of the figures call out as well as our relating with the figures. There is, to me, a resonance with the figures.

KAY: Because the figures are there, you mean?

MARIA: Because they're there and they're alive and they've been used over and over again. Sometimes I think that the figures call out to us as well as our relating to the figures. There seems to be a resonance in and with the figures.

KAY: It does have this feeling. That's the reason I liked having a separate room from the consult room. But I had never thought of it that way. However, when I think back, what you are both saying is true. Opening that door, going in – I called it my nonverbal room – the essence of the room carries with it – what do we use? – the word "spiritual." The room takes on a numinosity in itself.

LUCIA: It does.

MARIA: That's right. That's it. And there's a numinous transference to the room and the figures for us, as well as for the sandplayer.

LUCIA: That's fascinating, though, because what we are talking about is that the experience of the sand room may be like when you walk into some of those great cathedrals in Europe and it's there – the experience of the numinous! You don't have to be a religious person. There's something there.

KAY: Or it is like walking into a forest.

LUCIA: Yes.

MARIA: It is because the very act of playing in the sand, the whole process, imbues the room with this experience. The figures are not just little figurines. The figurines have been used over and over again and are alive with their own energy.

KAY: Are you saying that even before a new person uses the sand, the figures may have a numinosity for that person because they've been used so many times?

MARIA: Exactly! And they're imbued with something that we all feel. And they call to us.

LUCIA: But how does that happen, Maria?

MARIA: That's the mystery. That's the numinosity.

KAY: The figures themselves have something in them because they've been used so many times. We all have had experiences like this.

MARIA: Sandplay therapists who work with kids in a school or an agency have reported to me that during one day there's often a theme that gets created. No child ever sees what the kid before them has made, but on a given day there will be a circus theme and the next day a farm theme, etc. It is like there's a resonance about those figures.

KAY: Like when there's a figure on your shelves that no one has used for a long time, and then someone comes in one morning and uses it and the rest of the day more people use it.

MARIA: That's it, that same thing.

LUCIA: What is that?

KAY: All of us have experienced it.

MARIA: That's the numinosity. The psyche is alive.

KAY: Right. It's real.

MARIA: The psyche has its own life that calls to us and we respond to it.

LUCIA: So the psyche has an energy of its own – which is present. It is a living thing.

KAY: It's a reality.

MARIA: That's right – the reality of the psyche.

KAY: A similar thing happens in verbal analysis. Someone will come in and talk about a certain thing and then maybe the next person comes in and talks about the same thing or notes a picture on the wall that the previous person had commented on. It's a mystery. One can't believe it until one has experienced it.

LUCIA: The sandplay set-up is made up of physical things: the toys and the sand, the room and the chairs. But the numinous is – I was going to say the numinous is something else, but it isn't. It is more but it includes the objects.

KAY: It's deeper than the objects.

MARIA: It's not just the objects? It's not just the material objects. It's the objects imbued with the psyche, the objects imbued with the inner experience of the person who uses them.

KAY: In relationship to the therapist.

MARIA: It's the whole connection. It's your connection to the figures, as well as to all the other sandplayers who used them. So it's the material figures plus all of this other psychic energy that comes from the sandplay therapist and the sandplayers.

LUCIA: And it's specific. It's a blend of specific things. When I try to work with a client using someone else's collection, I find that I can hardly do it. The other therapist's figures, their sand, their room may be beautiful, but somehow it's –

KAY: You aren't connected enough with the energy yet.

MARIA: There's no numinosity for you!

LUCIA: What in the world? What is *numen*?

MARIA: *Numen* is the spirit or divine power and *pneuma* –

KAY: That comes from breath.

LUCIA: It's life. Isn't that the spirit of life?

MARIA: Spirit, breath – the breath of life.

LUCIA: Life. It's what God blows into Adam's nose.

KAY: In the mud – the mud of Adam.

MARIA: The material imbued with spirit or divine power. The figure has spirit!

LUCIA: There it is!

MARIA: Ah-ha. We got there. That was good. But we don't have to make it religious, we can refer to the Biblical story of Adam as a myth. But the connection is to spirit, and religion and spirit are connected, and God is part of the spirit.

LUCIA: Since the beginning of time – with fire and lightning – there has been the Great Spirit.

KAY: In all cultures.

MARIA: And indigenous peoples saw objects as imbued with life.

KAY: The idea that there is a spirit helps people to explain the mysteries of death and birth. And each culture has the same basic archetypes supposedly – but then they also have their culture and their experiences with their families.

LUCIA: So we're saying then, that – since the beginning – there was, it seems, some awareness in human beings of a living, vital energy of some kind. So what we are talking about is the numinous, God, spirit, the Self –

MARIA: Living spirit, psyche, the soul.

KAY: The trouble with using words is that you lose something. You can't put it into words.

MARIA: We're trying to get at something that is ineffable, so we are going to have a lot of words that are going to be used interchangeably and that's okay – because we're playing. The words are just fingers pointing – pointing at the moon. And since there are three of us, we'll have a lot of fingers. Although whatever "it" is, it is *not* the fingers pointing at the moon.

KAY: Granted it's difficult to use words but we're trying to get them together in a way that will communicate some of our experiences with the numinous and the spiritual, because we think it's valuable.

LUCIA: But didn't we just say that there is a mysterious place – experience – that words do not touch and sometimes destroy?

KAY: Right.

LUCIA: So we keep using this word "mystery" because, in the final analysis, we don't know what *it* is.

MARIA: It's a mystery. It's a mystery and, if we could know what *it* is, *it* wouldn't be a mystery.

LUCIA: It's inexplicable.

MARIA: Right. There it is. It's spirit. It's numinous. It's a mystery.

LUCIA: But it's living. I feel better when there's been some kind of a connection in the sand. Sometimes, if there's no sand and there's talk, I'm left a little bit troubled, unsettled. But if sandplayers do a tray and I experience the movement of the Self – of the numinous or whatever –

KAY: The energy of the Self.

LUCIA: I'm thinking of some of these television shows that are on now. It just amazes me – all this demon stuff and witches and all this stuff that's on TV. Now this is a weird combination if we're talking about God. But lately – I feel better. In some recent TV shows about magic, there is a magic formula or something that calls forth a force. There has to be a calling forth. There is an intention for both the dark forces and the light forces to come forth. I'm wondering in doing sandplay if we have to have an intention, a calling forth of that living, numinous energy.

KAY: [strikes a small Tibetan Buddhist bell]

LUCIA: There it is – the call! See, that's something that the Buddhists have – that is an intention.

KAY: Without words.

LUCIA: That's right. Now I, as the sandplay therapist, have to be in relationship with this energy, this intention. It's a calling. I think we call without consciously doing it.

MARIA: And again, you have to say, it isn't just we that call. The figures also call. The room calls. The whole relationship calls. Our experience of the calling calls.

LUCIA: But if we didn't hold that in our own psyches, the figures might not call.

MARIA: No, they would not call.

LUCIA: I don't think so. And the sand certainly wouldn't either. It's just a box of sand.

KAY: It's like pressing a button that opens up something in the communication.

LUCIA: They're just material figures unless the psyche of the therapist calls to God or to that living, numinous energy. Other cultures have rituals or there is an acknowledgment of the call. When you go into the priesthood, you are called.

KAY: Jungian analysts used to always talk about this. When I first became a Jungian analyst, I went to a meeting and they were all asking, "Now, how did you get the call?"

MARIA: I'm reading Jung's *Psychology and Religion*, in order to remember that call. Jung talks about the clergy and psychotherapists making that connection to the phenomena of the psyche, which is the living religious experience.

LUCIA: When I teach sandplay, someone may say, upon having an experience of the numinous through seeing a sandplay series, "This is what I wanted to do. Why I wanted to be a therapist. I knew there was something that I wanted to connect with, but nobody ever told me what it was, nobody ever talked about this before. But I knew that it was here." You see? That's the calling. That's why I like to teach, because I call for that in the students.

KAY: People who are suffering from stress or pain have something inside that knows what they need. The psyche reaches out for what it needs. The psyche has to know. You can't just go to a therapist to have a sandplay experience, I don't think, unless you have something that is directing you.

MARIA: The call.

LUCIA: Now, what calls? But why do some people respond to sandplay and some don't? So what happens when the spirit isn't moving?

KAY: We all have pain. We all have problems, but some of those things we can solve in some other way, a less expensive way. But if that doesn't solve it and the pain gets worse, then something happens and the psyche comes out and says, "Look, you've got to do something about this."

LUCIA: I wonder if that is connected to the – the fear. If you let go, if you cross into this place, your whole world is going to change.

KAY: And so it's an unknown.

LUCIA: And I don't want it to change.

KAY: Even though I'm in pain.

LUCIA: Change is more fearsome than the pain that I'm experiencing. So maybe that's where that fear of the Self comes in because the Self demands change. It will give you change.

KAY: And you can't go back.

LUCIA: No, you cannot go back. I've tried.

KAY: If you go through the gate, and you go on, it's all new. If you have your therapist with you, then it isn't so scary. And you can do it. And then you find out that this feels good. And then you can go through another gate.

MARIA: In sandplay we're taught that the experience of the Self and the experience of the numinous is an essential part of the sandplay work. I remember Kay's saying once, "People suffer, but then if they have an experience of the Self or the numinous, it's essential and it could change their life. When we are suffering, an experience of the numinous gives us something to hold onto." At that time I was in such a dark place myself, I was so glad you said that. You reminded me. You helped me remember. So thank you, Kay.

KAY: Aren't you dear!

MARIA: In order to go through the dark night of the soul, we need that connection to the numinous – and the spirit – to keep going. Sandplay and the sandplay therapist hold this space and possibility open for us.

LUCIA: I've always wondered about what was written over Jung's door, "Called or not called . . ."

KAY: Of course, it's in Latin. It translates to, "Called or not called, God will be there."

MARIA: So doing sandplay connects us to the God who will be there.

KAY: It's such a relief.

Chapter 30

Numinous

Maria Ellen Chiaia

> But in the face of possession or violent emotion, reason is abrogated; the numinous archetype proves on occasion to be the stronger because it can appeal to a vital necessity . . . We know that an archetype can break with shattering force into an individual human life and into the life of a nation. It is therefore not surprising that it is called "God."
>
> (Jung, 1963, par. 787)

Jung describes the experience of an archetype as a numinous experience. In sandplay we, the therapists, hold a space open in the co-transference, where there is the possibility of connecting to the phenomenon of the psyche, which includes the experience of the "numinous archetype." As Jung states above, the phenomenon of the psyche is an experience that is beyond consciousness and rational understanding, where consciousness loses its ascendancy.

In doing a sandplay the sandplayer is called by the sand, water and figures and responds to this calling not by rational responses, such as thinking and understanding, but by the inner feelings and responses evoked by the sand, water and figures. A resonance between the sandplayer and the sand, water and figures begins to happen. The sandplayer is called into action, picking the figures up or moving the sand around, and a sand picture is created. In doing a sandtray, the sandplayer may have an experience of the *numinosum*, "an experience of the subject independent of his will" (Jung, 1969a, par. 6). Jung states that something external to the individual causes this experience of the *numinosum* to happen.

Entering the sandplay room, with its sand, water and miniatures that have been used over and over again for this purpose, may feel like entering into liminal space, which is a threshold between ordinary reality and spiritual reality. This experience of external liminal space may call to the sandplayer and be felt as something independent from the sandplayer's will and control.

Jung goes on to say that "the *numinosum* is either a quality belonging to a visible object or the influence of an invisible presence that causes a peculiar alteration of consciousness" (1969a, par. 6). As discussed in the trialogues, the individual figures and/or the sandtray or the liminal space of the sandplay room may be felt as numinous and then there is the possibility for alteration of consciousness that Jung describes. I have always felt that when a sandplayer is creating a sandtray, often the sandplayer enters into an altered state of consciousness as they gain access to the unconscious and all of the possibilities for its expression. The sandplayer is moved by something that is beyond personal will and control, and then I am also moved as I experience what is emerging in the sandtray. Both of our consciousnesses are altered by this experience of the unconscious, as something not known has emerged and is being seen by the sandplayer and the therapist.

One of the definitions of "numinous" is being filled with the sense of the presence of divinity: holy. The sandplayer creating a sandplay enters into a realm of mystery and not knowing, and this may be felt as a living religious or holy experience. An ineffable awe may fill one as wonder, magic and spirit are felt and the presence of something larger than oneself becomes known. A sense of the light may change, radiating and reflecting a beauty and depth that is powerful and whole.

Some people, however, are afraid to surrender to such experiences for fear that they may be overtaken by strong feelings and become overwhelmed and/or frightened. They may have a "holy dread" of the numinous, a term that Jung borrowed from Rudolf Otto (Jung, 1969a, par. 222). Jung states:

> The "holy dread" of civilized man differs but little from the awe of the primitive, and that God who is present and active in the mystery is a mystery to both.
>
> (1969a, par. 375)

So sandplay can be frightening and overwhelming, and the calming empathic presence of the therapist who has experienced this process is essential.

Many feelings are generated in a sandplayer and the therapist. The ego may feel small and relative in the face of these powerful emotions as fear and loathing fill a person. In a sandtray, God may appear as a fierce image of the suffering Christ or the crucifixion, a witch, a large snake or shark, or dogs from hell. Or God may appear when quietness, trust, calm, peacefulness, wholeness or awe is present and there is an experience of being held in and by something larger than oneself. In this case, the Madonna, Buddha, saints, gods and goddesses or deities from different religions may be used. A God image can also be created from objects such as marbles, rocks, shells or driftwood, which create a pattern (Figure 30.1), or a shape created in the sand may reflect God in nature, God as part of the earth (Figure 30.2). Jung states:

> God-images carry ... an extraordinary numinosity. The tremendous effectiveness (*mana*) of these images is such that they not only give one the feeling of pointing to God but make one convinced that they actually

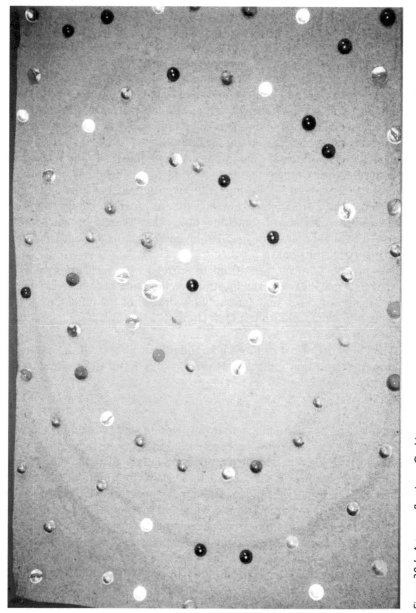

Figure 30.1 A tray reflecting a God image

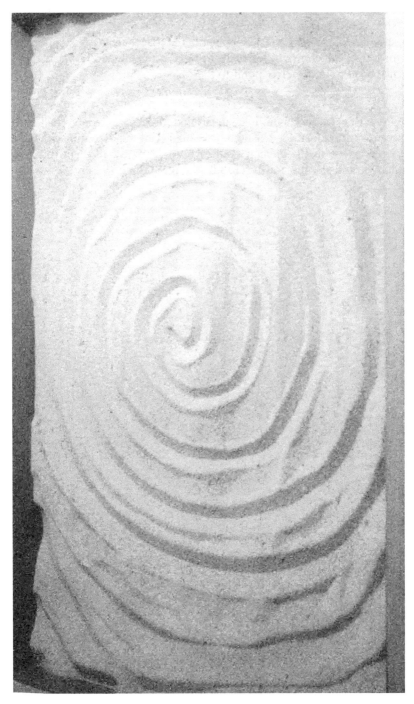

Figure 30.2 A tray reflecting God in nature

express and establish it as a fact ... It is, in fact, impossible to demon-
strate God's reality to oneself except by using images which have arisen
spontaneously ... it must be remembered that the images ... are psychic
processes which are different from their transcendental object; they do
not posit it, they merely point to it.

(1969a, par. 358)

Jung describes individuation as a psychic process in which real nature
transcends consciousness. The numinous quality of individuation can be seen
and experienced in the created sandtrays. In sandplay, through the images
that have arisen spontaneously, God is seen and God is present.

Chapter 31

Numinous

Kay Bradway

The word "numinous" was introduced into writings in the field of psychology by Rudolph Otto in the 1920s. Lionel Corbett later wrote that Otto had coined the word by combining the Latin word *numen*, meaning a god, with the verb *nuere*, meaning to nod or beckon, the combination indicating divine approval (Otto, 1958, pp. 6–7; Corbett, 1996, p. 11). The concept of "the numinous" has proved difficult to talk about or write about because, as has been stated a thousand times, it is not describable in words. In attempts to find words to identify a numinous experience, we say mystery, the unknown, magical, essence, connection with the Self, sacred, spiritual.

Appreciation for, and understanding of, the numinous and spiritual have been furthered by some of Jung's concepts such as synchronicity, archetypes, universal unconscious. The connection between the conscious and the universal unconscious may provide for mental telepathy or numinous connections between people.

David Feinstein offers the concept of "subtle energy" as a possible key in understanding what happens in numinous and spiritual experiences. He points to the universality of the recognition of such experiences by noting the many cultures that have a name or concept "to describe energies or fields that cannot be experienced directly through the senses yet are believed to influence people's lives." The names include *Ch'i* in countries using acupuncture, *ki* in Japan, *prana* in India and Tibet, *haraka* in Sufism, *waken* in the Lakota Sioux tradition, *menghe* in the pygmy culture of the Northeastern Congo forests, and *yesod* in the Jewish Kabbalistic tradition (Feinstein, 2003, p. 21).

Feinstein suggests that "Subtle energies may also prove to be a link between life in a physical body and nature's archetypal or spiritual realms" (2003, p. 35).

The need for the naming of experiences is bypassed in sandplay therapy. Verbal communication is replaced by a viewing together of visual images, obviating the need for names. Sandplay not only provides the space for the numinous/spiritual to occur and be developed; it also provides for the simultaneous viewing and experiencing of it by the client and therapist. In most complete processes, we clearly see the accessing of the spiritual, regardless of a client's religious beliefs. Joel Ryce-Menuhin writes, "Many agnostics and atheists have discovered through sandplay the unconscious release of integrative archetypal material which consciously enables them to contact the god image within their own psyche" (1992, p. 104).

In reviewing the processes of the sandplayers who worked with me, I found that most had actively experienced the spiritual in their process. This occurs in many different ways. Some clients entered sandplay with a wish to connect with the spiritual, consciously seeking it in their trays. Other clients were directed by their psyches to the spiritual despite their conscious attempt to steer clear of spiritual images. A few examples follow.

In her initial tray Rhoda presented the spiritual in the form of a glass sphere on a silver coil with, as she said, "powerful forces guarding the spiritual." She explained that the spiritual had always been there for her but she had lost touch with it. Her baby daughter with whom she was having problems at that time became the source of her experiencing the living spiritual as a mother. In the course of her process, she reconnected with the spiritual through working out her problems with her daughter.

Debbie, on the other hand, initially voiced distaste for using Christian images. Toward the end of making her first tray, she put in a Madonna and said, "I'm suspicious of Christian symbols but somehow something made me put it in." Debbie had come to do sandplay in order to prepare herself for her death, which her physician had told her would occur within the next two years. Somehow she knew that sandplay would help her get through this fateful period. Her connection with the spiritual persisted, in some form, throughout most of the trays. It was as if in this critical time her psyche, her Self, guided her placements in the tray in such a way that she not only accepted, but eventually embraced, the spiritual. In her final tray she highlighted the Madonna by standing her on a crescent moon. This seemed to give her the spiritual strength she required to meet her inevitable death. She died with serenity and without pain.

Emmy had stayed clear of religion ever since her mother had, as she said, "threatened" her with it as a child. In her initial tray, after it seemed completed, she casually tossed a couple of stones into the lower left. Later I realized that these stones must have represented, as rocks do in both primitive and Christian religions, the image of the gods. I came to believe that in this way they represented the unwanted and partly repressed and denied need to live out a more spiritual part of herself. In our review, Emmy recalled that a month after making this scene she had attended a Bach festival which represented the beginning of her search to find a renewed connection with a church. In her final scene one of the initial-tray stones that had been tossed aside was placed in a central position at the bottom. In our review she recalled that one month after this final scene she had gone to an Easter service for the first time since as a child she had spurned all religious experiences because of her mother's "threat."

In Ida's sandplay process she repeated a portrayal of the "sacred pool" over a period of many months. This finally brought her up out of the darkness to psychic healing. In one session she portrayed a leaving of the "sacred pool." But it was premature and she returned to it for the next several sessions. She appeared to need this long, safe protection of the sacred before she could deal with the wounds that she had experienced in connection with a previous damaging religious experience.

Ilsa was referred by her analyst for sandplay with me as a method that might go deeper and connect her with some vital spiritual space to help her get over her decreased energy. I have found that connecting or reconnecting with the spiritual is what is needed in instances of decreased energy and depression. In Ilsa's initial tray she presented several indications of touching into the deeper layers of her unconscious: the world egg, a silvered tree, colored glass pellets that she called "jewels." In her second tray there was evidence that she was descending further. The most significant themes in this tray included the protective male god Jizo and a Central American god looking over the whole scene. As with Rhoda, mothering was a prominent and necessary accompaniment to the spiritual journey. It was after Ilsa included an image of mother–child unity in her third tray that she used the beaded snake to represent something spiritual. In her fourth tray the Self was manifested: a centering pine emerging from a round shell with the male god Jizo and the white spiritual horse looking on. Treasures previously buried were now in full view. When this scene was presented on the screen at the review attended by the referring analyst, the analyst quietly commented, "It sends goose bumps up and down my spine" – a trustworthy evidence of the numinous in a Self tray.

Ursula, who made just ten trays in fifteen years, represented the connection with the spiritual after a tray that was experienced as a Self tray. Ursula had a punishing animus. She constantly criticized herself for everything – her choice in carpeting, the giving of parties, her poetry (which I found good), but mostly for the raising of her adopted child. It was only after I ceased pointing out her successes, in an attempt to counteract her negative feelings, that she, or rather her inner guide, helped her to get out of the negative place. She made a scene in the tray in which a figure representing herself was blocked from entering a sacred temple. She included a female figure who was looking on with compassion but not attempting to help (her therapist?). In making the next scene Ursula presented the figure of herself as gaining entrance to the sacred temple. In our later review of her completed sandplay process, she reported she had put in two guardians to protect her way and that she was then able to make her way safely to the sacred temple. She reported a feeling of release after this tray. She said that she had gained access to all the temples and all belonged to her. She had truly achieved access to the spiritual, the numinous, the sacred, the Self – the thing with the many names and no name.

Chapter 32

Numinous

Lucia Chambers

Vocatus atque non vocatus deus aderit.

Jung was frequently asked about a Latin inscription carved in stone over the doorway of his home. It translates as, "Invoked or not invoked the god will be present" (1977, p. 453). He explained when asked about it that he "wanted to express the fact I always feel unsafe, as if I am in the presence of superior possibilities" (p. 258). He said that it was a statement of the truth that he had experienced in his lifetime. "Religious phenomena are to be met everywhere," he said, "whether they are intentional or not" (p. 453). In a letter written in 1945, Jung states:

> The main interest of my work is not concerned with the treatment of neurosis but rather with the approach to the numinous. But the fact is that the approach to the numinous is the real therapy and inasmuch as you attain the numinous experiences you are released from the curse of pathology.
>
> (1973, p. 377)

Jung borrowed the word *numinous* from the work of Rudolf Otto to designate "the essence of holiness, or religious experience – in the presence of which is a *mystery* inexpressible and above all human creatures" (Jung, 1977, p. 453). Beyond the personal life experiences of pain, trauma, despair and anger, which afflict all humankind, there is a larger consciousness or a greater reality. This greater energy cannot be managed, directed or controlled because it pushes its way directly from our unconscious. It has an intentionality to gather together the bits and pieces of our fractured totality and bring them into a unified entity. When this happens, we experience the *numinosum*, the divine mystery. Corbett calls this an "incarnation of Self" (1996, p. 133); Dora Kalff called it a "manifestation of the Self" (1980, p. 29). Jung said it "provides a quality of experience which is synonymous with what has always been considered the religious domain" (Corbett, 1996, p. 9). Hillman says that "Depth psychology is thoroughly involved a priori with religion because it is a psychology of the soul . . . psychology does not take place without religion, because there is always a God in what we are doing" (1976, p. 228).

Many religious practices and rituals have to do with calling forth that experience of the *numinosum*. Prayer, meditation, ceremonies, incantations, fragrances, music and sometimes painful body postures are all efforts at summoning the divine experience. Sometimes we are given the experience, and sometimes we are not. That choice is not determined by our conscious self. This is why there is the mystery, the Divine Mystery.

We, in sandplay, also try to summon the experience of the "other" dimension by providing a space, the free and protected space. Perhaps we believe that if we build a field, they will come; a field free of limitations, expectations and reason. Sandplay therapists hold the open space, sustained by their own experience with the mystery; and the client, with great courage, sustained by the steady presence of the therapist, moves toward the unknown. Sometimes there is an experience of the numinous and sometimes there is not! But when the God-image does come, or the Self manifests, both client and therapist are fundamentally changed.

It is only through our experience that we can meet this other reality, not through the intellect but on a visceral level. There is an affective intensity. We might sense a warm wave of peace, an overwhelming awe, an upsurge of joy, a sudden eruption of tears or trembling, or a sense of the stopping of time. There is an energy present that moves both the client and the therapist into the totality which is the essence of life. Life then takes on a meaning and significance that it did not have before. A numinous experience forever changes us in ways that we can neither comprehend nor control. We are "seized" (Corbett, 1996, p. 17).

As Hillman believes, everyone comes with a calling. The calling is sometimes ignored, forgotten, and not understood. But it possesses you. And it will claim you. It does not go away (1976).

If we forget that we have been seized by a greater power and our egos begin to claim the ability to control and manipulate the mystery, we have been claimed by hubris, a spiritual inflation. It is then inevitable that we will be brought low: as Icarus crashed to earth when he devalued the power of the sun, so too will our egos be shattered as we are grounded into suffering.

All religious mythologies recognize that creation emerges out of undifferentiated base, dark matter or *mater*. The shining lotus emerges from primordial ooze, the golden phoenix rises from the ashes of its cremation, Christ appears risen from the darkness of his tomb. The great Gothic cathedrals that soar upward in unbelievable loftiness have images of Black Madonnas in the dark of the crypts beneath their stone floors, and dank-smelling wells there sink deep into the earth. Soul making, or the realigning with the Self, always involves a going back down into the *prima materia* and therefore is always a defeat for the ego and can promote an experience of suffering. The ego must be broken down and shattered because it has become too centralized and confining. The imagination has dried up and life's meaning has become shallow or nonexistent. The ego will struggle to defend itself. There will be denial, massive projections and maybe a clinical depression. Perhaps medication will then be used to alleviate the psychological pain that comes when the gods demand their rightful place. No sooner will one hole in the defenses against change be shored up than the Self will very often break through from another quarter, many times in the very place where we have built our highest and strongest protection: protection against the demands of the gods to enter. The Self demands entrance and our resistance becomes our suffering. Personal suffering always carries within it an aspect of the divine. When we can acknowledge that the pain we are experiencing is not arbitrary, but is actually a call to move us toward a reality of greater dimension, we can diminish the tendency to identify with the suffering, and pathologize ourselves and be "sick." We have the conscious opportunity to recognize that what we are experiencing is the longing within the human soul for a reunion with itself. Perhaps we can yield and join in the search.

> The decisive question for us is, "Are we related to Something Infinite or not?" That, I would suggest, is the explicit foundation of the work that we do.
>
> (Ulanov, 1999, p. 159)

References

Abram, D. (1996) *The Spell of the Sensuous*, New York: Vintage Books.

Abrams, J. and Zeig, C. (eds) (1991) *Meeting the Shadow*, New York: St Martin's Press.

Allan, J. (1988) *Inscapes of the Child's World*, Dallas, TX: Spring Publications.

Bair, D. (2003) *Jung, a Biography*, Boston, MA: Little, Brown & Company.

Balint, M. (1999) *The Basic Fault: Therapeutic Aspects of Regression*, London: Routledge.

Barnhart, C.L. (ed.) (1947) *American College Dictionary*, Toronto: Random House.

Baum, L.F. (1956) *The Wizard of Oz*, New York: Del Rey Books/Ballantine Books; first published 1900.

Beebe, J. (1992) *Integrity in Depth*, College Station, TX: A&M University Press.

—— (2003) "What is the Self?", a talk by John Beebe, Analytical Psychology Club of San Francisco.

Berry, P. (ed.) (1990) *Fathers and Mothers*, Dallas, TX: Spring Publications.

Bradway, K. (1982) *Villa of Mysteries: Pompeii Initiation Rites of Women*, San Francisco, CA: The C.G. Jung Institute of San Francisco.

—— (2001) "What is sandplay and how does it work?", Presentation Division 39 of Psychoanalysis of the American Psychological Association, 21st Annual Spring Meeting, Santa Fe, NM.

—— (2004) "Purposeful imaging," *Journal of Sandplay Therapy*, **13**, 2: 6–9.

Bradway, K. and Feldman, B. (2002) "Child analysis using Kalff and Fordham," *Journal of Sandplay Therapy*, **11**, 1: 43–49.

Bradway, K. and McCoard, B. (1997) *Sandplay – Silent Workshop of the Psyche*, New York: Routledge.

Buber, M. (1958) *I and Thou*, New York: Charles Scribner & Sons.

Cameron, S. (2001) "Recognizing the appearance of the Self in sandplay therapy," Dissertation, The California School of Professional Psychology at Alameda.

Chambers, L. (1990) "The inturning spiral: The path to the healing of the feminine," *Northern California Sandplay Society Newsletter*, fall.

Chiaia, M.E. (1995) "A modern day rite," *Journal of Sandplay Therapy*, **4**, 2: 75–88.

—— (1996) "The seed of life: Birth of a woman and a child," *Journal of Sandplay Therapy*, **5**, 2: 88–111.

—— (1997) *Imagination in Dialogue*, Ann Arbor, MI: UMI Dissertation Services.

Chiaia, M. and Grand, I.J. (2002) "On not killing the mystery: Imagination in sandplay research," *In the Hands of Creation: Sandplay Images of Birth and Rebirth*, eds Baum, N. and Weinberg, B., Toronto: Muki Baum Association.

Cirlot, J.E. (1982) *A Dictionary of Symbols*, New York: Philosophical Library.

Cooper, J.C. (1988) *An Illustrated Encyclopedia of Traditional Symbols*, London: Thames & Hudson.

Corbett, L. (1996) *The Religious Function of the Psyche*, New York and London: Routledge.

Crichton, M. (1990) *Jurassic Park*, New York: Ballantine Books.

Eliade, M. (1976) *Myths, Rites, Symbols*, Vol. 1, eds Doty, W.G. and Beanne, W.C., New York: Harper & Row.

Feinstein, D. (2003) "Subtle energy: Psychology's missing link," *Ions Noetic Sciences Review*, **64**: 18.

Fierz-David, L. (1988) *Women's Dionysian Initiation*, Dallas, TX: Spring Publications.

Fordham, M. (1970) *Children as Individuals: An Analytical Psychologist's Study of Child Development*, New York: C.P. Putnam's Sons.

Grand, I.J. (1999) *Collaboration and Creativity: An Interdisciplinary Study*, Ann Arbor, MI: UMI Dissertation Services.

Hall, J.A. (1983) *Jungian Dream Interpretation – A Handbook of Theory and Practice*, Toronto: Inner City Books.

Hedges, L. (1994) *Working the Organizing Experience: Transforming, Psychotic, Schizoid, and Autistic States*, Northvale, NJ: Jason Aronson.

Henderson, J.L. (1967) *Thresholds of Initiation*, Middletown, CT: Wesleyan University Press.

—— (1990) *Shadow and Self*, Wilmette, IL: Chiron Publications.

Hesse, H. (1976) *Demian*, Catchoque, NY: Buccaneer Publishers.

Hillman, J. (1972) *The Myth of Analysis*, Evanston, IL: Northwestern University Press.

—— (1976) *Re-visioning Psychology*, New York: Harper & Row.

Jacoby, M. (1999) *Jungian Psychotherapy and Contemporary Infant Research: Basic Patterns of Emotional Exchange*, London and New York: Routledge.

Jaffe, A. (1972) *From the Life and Work of C.G. Jung*, translated by R.F.C. Hull, London: Hodder & Stoughton.

Johnson, B. (1988) *Lady of the Beasts*, New York: Harper & Row.

Jones, R. (1937) *Christian Faith and Practice in the Experience of Friends*, London: Yearly Meeting Publication.

Jung, C.G. (1933) *Modern Man in Search of a Soul*, Florida: Harcourt Brace & Co.

—— (1953) *Two Essays on Analytical Psychology, Collected Works*, 7, New York: Bollingen Foundation.

—— (1959) *AION: Researches into the Phenomenology of the Self, Collected Works*, 9, Part 2, 2nd edn, Princeton, NJ: Princeton University Press.

—— (1960) *Answer to Job*, Cleveland, OH: World Publishing.

—— (1963) *Mysterium Coniunctionis, Collected Works*, 14, Princeton, NJ: Princeton University Press.

—— (1966a) *Two Essays on Analytical Psychology, Collected Works*, 7, Princeton, NJ: Princeton University Press.

—— (1966b) *The Spirit in Man, Art, and Literature, Collected Works*, 15, Princeton, NJ: Princeton University Press.

—— (1966c) *The Practice of Psychotherapy, Collected Works*, 16, Princeton, NJ: Princeton University Press.

—— (1966d) *Psychology of the Transference, Collected Works*, 16, Princeton, NJ: Princeton University Press.

—— (1968a) *Psychology and Alchemy, Collected Works*, 12, Princeton, NJ: Princeton University Press.

—— (1968b) *The Archetypes and the Collective Unconscious, Collected Works*, 9, Part 1, Princeton, NJ: Princeton University Press.

—— (1968c) *Alchemical Studies, Collected Works*, 13, Princeton, NJ: Princeton University Press.

—— (1969a) *Psychology and Religion: West and East, Collected Works*, 11, 2nd edn, Princeton, NJ: Princeton University Press.

—— (1969b) *The Structure and Dynamics of the Psyche, Collected Works*, 8, Princeton, NJ: Princeton University Press.

—— (1969c) *Psychological Factors in Human Behaviour, Collected Works*, 8, Princeton, NJ: Princeton University Press.

—— (1970) *Psychological Reflections*, eds Jacobi, J. and Hull, R.F.C., Princeton, NJ: Princeton University Press.

—— (1973) *Letters*, Vol. 1, eds Adler, G. and Jaffe, A., Princeton, NJ: Princeton University Press.

—— (1977) *C.G. Jung Speaking*, McGuire & Hall (eds), Princeton, NJ: Princeton University Press.

—— (1979) *Word and Image*, ed. Jaffe, A., Princeton, NJ: Princeton University Press.

Jung, C.G. and Kerenyi, C. (1973) *Essays on the Science of Mythology*, Princeton, NJ: Bollingen Series/Princeton University Press.

Kalff, D.M. (1980) *Sandplay, a Psychotherapeutic Approach to the Psyche*, Santa Monica, CA: Sigo Press.

—— (2003) *Sandplay, a Psychotherapeutic Approach to the Psyche*, new edn, Cloverdale, CA: Temenos Press.

Kalsched, D. (1996) *The Inner World of Trauma: Archetypal Defenses of the Personal Spirit*, New York: Routledge.

Kawai, H. (1996) *Buddhism and the Art of Psychotherapy*, College Station, TX: A&M University Press.

Kirsch, T. (2000) *The Jungians – A Comparative and Historical Perspective*, London: Routledge.

Kohut, H. (1993) *The Restoration of the Self*, Madison, CT: International Universities Press.

Lewis, T., Amini, F., and Lannon, R. (2001) *A General Theory of Love*, New York: Vintage Books.

Lowenfeld, M. (1979) *The World Technique*, London: George Allen & Unwin.

Macdonald, D. (ed.) (1987) *The Encyclopedia of Mammals*, New York: Facts on File Publications.

McLean, A. (1991) *A Commentary on the Mutus Liber*, Grand Rapids, MI: Phanes Press.

Maier, M. (1989) *Atalanta Fugiens*, trans. & ed. Goodwin, J., Grand Rapids, MI: Phanes Press.

Milner, M. (1969) *The Hands of the Living God*, New York: International Universities Press.

Mitchell, R. and Friedman, H. (1994) *Sandplay: Past, Present and Future*, London: Routledge.

Mitchell, S. (1993) *Hope and Dread in Psychoanalysis*, New York: Basic Books/Harper Collins.

Moore, T. (1992) *Care of the Soul*, New York: Harper Collins.

Neumann, E. (1963) *The Great Mother, an Analysis of the Archetype*, Princeton, NJ: Princeton University Press.

—— (1964) *The Origins and History of Consciousness*, New York: Bollingen.

—— (1973) *The Child, Structure and Dynamics of the Nascent Personality*, New York: G.P. Putnam's Sons.

Otto, R. (1958) *The Idea of the Holy*, Oxford: Oxford University Press.

The Oxford Dictionary of 20th Century Quotations (1998) New York: Oxford University Press.

Peck, M.S. (1983) *People of the Lie*, New York: Simon & Schuster.

Pirsig, R.M. (1974) *Zen and the Art of Motorcycle Maintenance*, London: The Bodley Head.

Richards, M. (1962) *Centering in Pottery, Poetry and the Person*, Littletown, CT: Wesleyan University Press.

Rilke, R.M. (1962) *Sonnets to Orpheus*, trans. Herter, M.D., New York: W.W. Norton.

Rosen, D. (1996) *The Tao of Jung*, New York: Penguin Books.

Rumi (1995) *The Essential Rumi*, New York: Harper Collins Publishing.

Ryce-Menuhin, J. (1992) *Jungian Sandplay: The Wonderful Therapy*, London: Routledge.

St. Exupery, A. (1943) *The Little Prince*, trans. Woods, K., San Diego and New York: Harvest/Harcourt Brace & Co.

Samuels, A. (1985) *Jung and the Post-Jungians*, London: Routledge & Kegan Paul.

Schwartz-Salant, N. (1995a) *Jung on Alchemy*, Princeton, NJ: Princeton University Press.

—— (1995b) "On the interactive field in analysis," *The Interactive Field in Analysis*, Wilmette, IL: Chiron.

—— (1998) *The Mystery of Human Relationship*, New York: Routledge.

Signell, K. (1991) *Wisdom of the Heart*, New York: Bantam Books.

—— (1996) "Silence and sandplay," *Journal of Sandplay Therapy*, **5**, 2: 68–87.

Silverman, L. (1985) "Mommy and I are one," *American Psychologist*, **40**, Dec., 12, 1296–1308.

Stein, M. (1982) *Jungian Analysis*, La Salle, IL: Open Court.

—— (1995a) *Jungian Analysis*, 2nd edn, Chicago, IL: Open Court.

—— (1995b) *The Interactive Field in Analysis*, Wilmette, IL: Chiron.

Stern, D. (1985) *The Interpersonal World of the Infant: A View from Psychoanalysis and Developmental Psychology*, New York: Basic Books.

Stevenson, R.L. (1944) *A Child's Garden of Verses*, Special Edition, New York: Heritage Press.

Ulanov, A. (1999) *Religion and the Spiritual in Carl Jung*, Mahwah, NJ: Paulist Press.

von Franz, M.L. (1972) *On Dreams and Death*, Boston, MA: Shambhala.

Von Keyserlingk, L. (1992) *Verwurzelt in Zimmer der Mutter der Mutter*, Rieden: Conpress Medienproduktion.

Walker, B.G. (1983) *The Woman's Encyclopedia of Myths and Secrets*, San Francisco, CA: Harper & Row.

Weinrib, E.L. (1983) *Images of the Self: The Sandplay Therapy Process*, Boston, MA: Sigo Press.

Winnicott, D.W. (1965) *The Maturational Processes and the Facilitating Environment:*

Studies in the Theory of Emotional Development, Madison, CT: International University Press.

—— (1986) *Playing and Reality*, London and New York: Tavistock Publications.

Wordsworth, W. (1943) *Wordsworth*, Cambridge: Penguin Books.

Young-Bruehl, W. and Bethelard, F. (2000) *Cherishment, a Psychology of the Heart*, New York: The Free Press.

Young-Eisendrath, P. (1997) *Gender and Desire*, College Station, TX: A&M University Press.

Index

T - #0023 - 101024 - C8 - 234/156/13 [15] - CB - 9781583917299 - Gloss Lamination